THE TRAVELER'S
NATURAL MEDICINE KIT

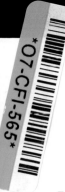

THE TRAVELER'S NATURAL MEDICINE KIT

Easy and Effective Remedies for Staying Healthy on the Road

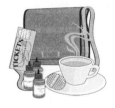

PAMELA HIRSCH

Healing Arts Press
Rochester, Vermont

Healing Arts Press
One Park Street
Rochester, Vermont 05767
www.InnerTraditions.com

Healing Arts Press is a division of Inner Traditions International

Note to the reader: This book is intended as an informational guide. The remedies, approaches, and techniques described herein are meant to supplement, and not to be a substitute for, professional medical care or treatment. They should not be used to treat a serious ailment without prior consultation with a qualified health care professional.

Library of Congress Cataloging-in-Publication Data

Hirsch, Pamela

   The traveler's natural medicine kit : easy and effective remedies for staying healthy on the road / Pamela Hirsch.

      p. cm.

   Includes bibliographical references.

   ISBN 0-89281-947-2 (paper)

   1. Travel—Health aspects. 2. Alternative medicine. 3. Herbs—Therapeutic use. 4. Self-care, Health. I. Title.

RA783.5 .H56 2001

613.6'8—dc21

                                                                2001016894

Printed and bound in Canada

10 9 8 7 6 5 4 3 2 1

Text design by Crystal H. H. Roberts

Layout by Rachel Goldenberg

This book was typeset in Granjon with Nueva as the display typeface

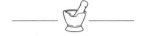

*To my grandfather, George Lee Kishlar, green man,
who taught me the ways of the Heart and respect
for all of Nature . . .*

*To my son, Robert, miracle child,
who taught me about Joy and of healing the Self . . .*

*To my husband, Duffy, true companion,
who always said I'd write books someday . . .*

*. . . this book is dedicated with love, respect,
and gratitude.*

CONTENTS

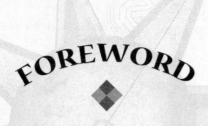

FOREWORD

WHETHER SOLITARY ADVENTURERS OR RIDERS in a caravan, travelers were once thought to be the bravest citizens of the world. Often risking their lives, they might journey through the jungle to the next village or across seas and deserts to a new world. When they returned, these adventurers were revered for the new knowledge they brought home. Travelers shared stories as well as samples of new foods, spices, and medicines. Sometimes they brought seeds, and these new delights were incorporated into the village lifestyle. Travelers were the doors to the outside world.

Today, of course, traveling is much more commonplace and certainly not our only means of cultural exchange. But exotic places still conjure up romantic visions of adventure, and even the most sophisticated traveler faces health-compromising dangers. Subjecting ourselves to new climes, germs, and foods, we introduce our bodies to stress and new types of intestinal flora, which we each process in our own unique way. Thank goodness Pam has written this book to help you prepare for the health issues that can and do come up on even the most well-planned trip.

Having read many books on natural medicine and self-healing in my twenty-eight years as an herbalist and educator, I was pleased to read this most honest and practical book. Knowing Pam personally, I see in this book her meticulous research and attention to detail. Pam draws on her extensive experience as a world traveler and a healer, sharing her successes and her mistakes and offering not just her personal wisdom but also the knowledge given to her by teachers and friends. I especially appreciate Pam's acknowledgment of the role attitude and spirit play in healing as we navigate life's many adventures.

In the modern world we now face complex viral diseases and bacteria resistant to pharmaceutical antibiotics. Many people believe the answer to this problem lies in a return to healthy living and natural remedies. Bacteria has a difficult time building a resistance to the complex chemical makeup of herbal remedies, and immune-enhancing foods and herbs allow us to become more resilient to viral infections. This book introduces to the reader, in a safe and simple way, the joys and benefits of natural self-healing. By applying these time-honored remedies, the reader is helping to keep alive ancient traditions and perhaps resolving some of the new problems we have created in our modern world.

In my personal travels, I always carry a small kit similar to the one recommended by Pam in this book. At the end of my trip, it is usually depleted not only from my own needs, but also from those of my fellow travelers. Often a successful remedy sparks a new friendship and plants the seeds of interest in this wonderful form of healing. I predict this book will become a favorite in homes desiring self-sufficiency, where it will be used not just for travel, but also as a home first-aid guide. I intend to keep my copy in a handy place.

Shatoiya de la Tour,
coauthor of *The Herbalist's Garden*

ACKNOWLEDGMENTS

MY LIFE HAS BEEN BLESSED WITH CARING friends, loving relatives, and more than a few "angels" who watch over me. A number of them have helped with the birth of this book. First, I want to thank Lee Juvan, my editor at Inner Traditions, who first proposed this book and is one of the most diplomatic people I know. I am delighted to call her my friend. Shatoiya de la Tour has not only been my herbal mentor, but a grandmother, mother, and sister rolled into one— a true wise woman. Thank you, Shatoiya.

Many of us would not have had the chances we've had if not for Rosemary Gladstar. She has selflessly given her knowledge to many of us and her life to the Green Nations. Thank you, Rosemary.

I want to thank Lois Johnson, M.D., who daily puts into practice the oath she took as a physician, for her excellent teachings and for completing the technical review of this book.

To my sister, Claudia Leavitt, who in many ways is the "spirit" of *Traveler's,* go my thanks. She was my traveling companion when we were younger and has always been my best friend, even when she didn't know it. I want to thank my parents, Margaret and Claude Hirsch. Without them, none of my travels would have been possible. It was my mother who lovingly taught me how to "make do" and my father who taught me that traveling is an opportunity in ambassadorship. I want to acknowledge and thank my grandfather George Lee Kishlar, who was my first teacher in the ways of all things green.

Thanks go to Mrs. Wally, my seventh grade English teacher, for teaching me to "write it just like you said it!" My thanks to the women of the Seasonal Circle, for your love and support during this past year. Thank you Brighid, for your inspiration and blessings.

Finally, I want to thank my son, Robbie, and my husband, Duffy, who always believed in my herbal work, have been excellent guinea pigs, and bless me every day with their love.

INTRODUCTION

TO PARAPHRASE CHARLES DICKENS, TRAVELING can be both the best of times and the worst of times. Often it's both—in one journey. Whether your trip is welcome or not, business or pleasure, it's almost always stressful. The planning, the anticipation, the mode of travel chosen, being away from home, plans gone awry, lack of sleep—all of these add up to stress. In the past three decades much has been published about the effects of stress, "good" and "bad," on our health. So it's not surprising that something as uprooting, and as uplifting, as travel can often result in blips in an otherwise healthy life.

I was born in Venezuela, spent the first three years of my life there, and then began a series of moves to the United States, North Africa, the Middle East, Europe, the Pacific Rim, and finally back to the States when I was in my early twenties. Many of the places where my father's work took him were considered third world, and while basic medical and first-aid supplies were generally available, I believe the environments I grew up in

1

engendered a desire in me to make do and find ways of self-medicating as well as medicating those I lived with. I remember once making up a batch of hard candy and adding a few teaspoons of Vicks VapoRub to it before it cooled. Dropping the resulting mixture onto waxed paper, I proudly informed my younger sister—who just happened to have a sore throat—that sucking on one of these candies would cure her immediately. She did so and pronounced them miraculous, as a little sister should. I think it might have been several years later when I read the back of the Vicks jar and noted the warning not to ingest the product. Intent and suggestion can work wonders—truly. She lives to this day. (I don't suggest making these throat lozenges yourself!)

Part of growing up abroad meant that we traveled regularly and often long distances to exotic locations. My parents saw to it that both my sister and I were well drilled in travel preparation, and after a while we learned what to take with us and what to leave at home. We often found ourselves without the one thing that would fix a problem. That was when we began to learn to improvise. Since this is a book on natural remedies, I shouldn't tell you that early on I found Pepto-Bismol tablets quite useful when I was unable to sleep. It was our first night at our destination, with a seven-hour difference in time zones, and my sister and I were alone in a darkened hotel room. Downstairs the occasional train lumbered into an empty station; a bar around the corner played strains of George Harrison's "My Sweet Lord." Yellow and red lights flickered and peeked around the heavy hotel room curtains. It was 2:30 A.M. and I couldn't get to sleep. Pepto-Bismol worked for me then but when I think about it now, thirty years later, it was really the only thing my mother had to give me. Intent, and love, is sometimes everything.

This brings me to improvisation. I don't want to imply that natural remedies are mere substitutes for conventional treatment. They're often an appropriate choice, depending on the individual and the situation. But it's often the case that when you're traveling, you're limited in the amount of baggage and "stuff" you can carry along. This means it's a good thing if items in your travel first-aid kit can do double or even triple duty. This book makes no attempt to regale you with a vast number of alternative remedies. I'd rather tell you about ten that could be successfully used for all the ailments I'll discuss—but unfortunately that would be simplistic. My goal instead is to help you think ahead so you can be amply prepared, suggest remedies perhaps considered old fashioned that are easily found in remote areas, and finally to think "out of the box" about reasonable alternatives—really just educated improvisation.

GENERAL TIPS FOR HAPPY TRAILS

Whether or not it's your stated goal, it helps to think of travel as a growth opportunity. What's the saying? "Attitude is everything." Well, maybe not, but if you do come down with something while on the road, a positive outlook will facilitate the healing process. Rather than work yourself into a depression, try to ascertain how your experience might benefit you. Amazingly, I've seen travelers become irritated about the fact that things are done differently abroad. "In the States it's not like this!" Well, no, we're not in Kansas any longer, Toto, and why would you travel anyhow if everything was the same as where you came from? I don't mean to be insensitive to the inconvenience of being ill while traveling. It is indeed emotionally difficult to deal with pains and sickness when the adventures of travel beckon. But if you can embrace the concept that there are gems of wisdom—little lessons—in *all* that happens on our journeys in life, both figuratively and in fact, you might find your disappointment receding. To this point, I offer seven tips.

1. **Be prepared—plan ahead.** Think about what you'll be doing on your trip, what kinds of activities will be available, and what ailments you might have as a result. For instance, if you're going hiking, moleskin would be an excellent item to have packed. If you know your child is prone to motion sickness, pack ginger capsules. There's more about all this in chapter 5, Making a Traveler's Medicine Kit.

2. **Keep a healthy outlook.** This really refers to the comments I made at the beginning of this section. It also means not obsessing about things that could happen. My friend Shatoiya de la Tour once told me, "Worrying is praying for bad things to happen." It was an eye-opener for me.

3. **Intention is often everything.** Healing without strong intent—the focused desire to effect a certain outcome—is devoid of spirit; there can be no true healing without it. The "laying on of hands" is a perfect example. Many times I've seen a less-than-perfect remedy facilitate a cure, and I'm convinced that the intent of the healer was the catalyst. My point is that if the remedy you have in your kit isn't exactly what you might use at home, but it's similar and can be used with the same principles in mind (and you know it to be safe), try it and "make it so."

4. **Do what you can—allow your body to do the rest.** This is a simple principle. Once you've made the effort—washed the wound, applied disinfectant and bandage—relax. Your body truly will do the rest. One of the principles of naturopathic medicine is the "recognition and encouragement of the body's inherent healing abilities."

5. **What is your body telling you?** Illness is often your body's way of communication. It may be trying to tell you something. If you aren't practiced in being aware of what's going on in your body and ascertaining the cause, the process can at first feel like walking through mud. Persevere.

   Headaches are a good example and place to start. See if you can remember what you ate or were doing prior to the headache. Maybe being in crowded or congested areas is a precursor for you. Perhaps a smoky bar was the trigger. The obvious thing to do is leave, or refrain from doing what brought the problem on. Travel can be overwhelming—remember that it's okay and appropriate to rest when you've had enough.

6. **Live a little.** This is a preventive. Traveling, even when you're on business, is a time to glory in the beauty of Earth and the differences and similarities of her inhabitants. Find out what the "natives" do—then see if you might not like to do the same. Trust me when I say that there's a wonderful sense of freedom and belonging in relieving yourself in the Sierra Mountains—once you get over the logistics, of course!

7. **Remain flexible.** Being rigid in your beliefs and ideas of what an outcome should be is a setup for disappointment. And I'm convinced that the same rigidity causes a hardening in the structures of the body and restricts the flow of chi, or life

force, thereby creating an environment for illness. See if you can remain unattached to outcomes, allowing events to unfold as they will. This doesn't mean you don't plan or try to affect what happens; it just means be flexible.

More practically, a discussion on the contents of this book is warranted. I've attempted to include as many of the minor ailments that experience has shown me seem to plague travelers as possible. Each section contains some basic information about the problem, and then some suggestions about how to treat it. Remedies include five major alternative healing modalities— herbal therapy, aromatherapy, homeopathy, flower essences, and supplements. Each of these modalities, except supplements, is discussed individually as a precursor to the section on ailments. I've used the term *supplement* somewhat loosely in this book, as a catchall for vitamins, minerals, and other natural, non-pharmaceutical substances that have been proven or thought to enhance health. Examples include vitamin C, magnesium, and melatonin. Each of these subcategories is so large in scope that I've made no attempt to describe it fully here. The book, *Prescription for Nutritional Healing,* by James F. Balch, M.D., and Phyllis A. Balch is an excellent resource for more information on the subject. I've also included a discussion of making your own first-aid kit(s); a listing of resources and a glossary of terms are offered as well.

If you will be traveling with a child, be sure to consult an experienced herbalist before you leave home to determine which herbs are appropriate for children's special needs. Throughout the book, I mention a few very gentle remedies that are considered safe for children, but overall this book is geared toward adults—and some herbs that are quite safe for adults are not recommended for children's use. The safest rule of thumb is: if in doubt—don't!

One note of warning: Just because a treatment is natural doesn't mean it's safe. The word *natural* is overused these days, and means only that something isn't synthetic. There are a number of natural substances that are, in fact, toxic and should not be used. Sadly, as herbal products become more mainstream while good education on their usage remains scarce, a prevalent concept is that because something is herbal, it's natural and therefore safe to use. Nothing could be further from the truth. In general, herbs work more slowly than drugs and have smaller amounts of toxins in them. Some herbs, however, are very poisonous; hemlock and foxglove are just two. Having made that statement, I still believe that herbs are far safer than most manufactured drugs and have fewer side effects. But please make sure that you know what you're using and have ascertained its safety. While much of what is discussed in this book is safe, misuse could pose a health threat. I have noted any safety issues throughout the book, as appropriate.

1
HERBAL
PREPARATIONS

THERE ARE MANY WAYS TO ADMINISTER HERBAL preparations. Some lend themselves to travel; others are easier to use at home. Broadly speaking, botanical remedies fall into the following groups: teas, compresses and poultices, oils and salves, tinctures, liniments, capsules and pills, and syrups. Due to the recent resurgence of herbal medicine in this country, most of these preparations are now easily purchased. In many cases they are also easily produced at home, and basic instructions on doing so are provided here. In addition, there are a number of well-written books on the subject. If making your own herbal preparations is something you'd like to try, any of Rosemary Gladstar's books would be an excellent place to start. And Richo Cech, owner of Horizon Herbs, recently published *Making Plant Medicine,* which combines clear instructions for making herbal medicines with humorous stories about life on an herb farm. (See the bibliography for more information.)

TEAS

Teas have been used for thousands of years for both healing and pleasure. It would probably be more appropriate to use the terms *infusion* and *decoction,* since *tea* really refers to the black tea originally from Asia that became so popular in England in the eighteenth century. Still, you'll often hear the word *tea* used as a catchall for any plant infusion or decoction.

Infusions

Pouring hot water over plant material that is delicate in nature constitutes an infusion. This includes flowers, leaves, and stems—usually the aerial parts of the plant. The plant matter is allowed to steep in hot water for 5 to 15 minutes, depending on the strength required. Many herb books give guidelines on recommended infusion times, depending on the particular herb. David Hoffmann's *The New Holistic Herbal* is an excellent example of such a book. A rule of thumb for amounts and infusion times is to use 1 teaspoon of *dried* herb or 1 tablespoon of *fresh* herb to 1 cup of hot water, and allow it to steep for 10 minutes. If you're using several herbs, make up your herbal formula first and then add 1 teaspoon or 1 tablespoon of the mixture to the hot water. You can buy special tea balls, spoons, and nets to hold the herb(s) in your teacup while they're steeping. Cover the cup with a saucer while it's steeping to prevent the medicinal properties from evaporating.

Using the ratio of herb to water described above, it is also possible to make a cold infusion by placing the appropriate amount of plant material in a jar and pouring cool or room-temperature water over it. Allow the resulting mixture to sit overnight. Strain the herbs from the tea the following morning to use. You don't need to refrigerate the infusion during the night as long as you take it by the following day. You may wish to refrigerate any remaining tea after straining. It will keep for a day in this manner. This is a particularly useful method for making infusions, because it requires no heat. Heat will destroy some of an herb's properties, so this is less destructive. I have found cold infusions to be an excellent way to make a quart of nettle tea for the next day.

Either a hot or a cold infusion can be easily prepared on the road if you've planned ahead. It's easy enough to ask your waitperson or hotel staff for some hot water for tea. If you're camping, try making a solar infusion. The process is exactly the same as the one described for a cold infusion, but rather than letting the herbs sit overnight, place the covered jar in the sun. Your tea will be ready in two to eight hours, depending on the desired strength.

Decoctions

A decoction is similar to an infusion but involves simmering the herbs in water, usually for about 15 minutes. This process is used when you want to make a tea with some of the woody, more resinous parts of a plant such as its bark, roots, rhizomes, or seeds. While decoctions are probably less convenient to make while traveling than infusions, it's worthwhile understanding the difference between the two methods and why you'd use one over the other. And it's always possible that you might be in a location with stove or campfire at your disposal.

To make a decoction, place the desired amount of herb(s) in

a saucepan and cover with water. As with infusions, a general guideline is 1 teaspoon of *dried* herb or 1 tablespoon of *fresh* herb to 1 cup of water. Cover the pan and bring the mixture to a simmer for about 15 minutes. It's important the keep the pan covered during the simmering process so that all the herb's properties stay with the decoction. When done, strain the liquid into a cup or container.

I was taught to formulate herbal blends for teas so that a plant's aerial parts or flowers were not mixed with roots. How would you prepare such a mix—as a decoction or an infusion? There are times, however, when you'll want both bark and leaf tea, or some other composition. In this case you can make each separately—the bark as a decoction, the leaves as an infusion—and mix them together afterward. Another method is to heat the whole mixture together with water in a saucepan and then turn off the heat as soon as a simmer occurs.

COMPRESSES AND POULTICES

When I first began my study of herbal medicine, I always confused compresses and poultices—were they the same? Perhaps called compresses in the North and poultices down South? They are, in fact, different, and each is used for a slightly different problem.

Compresses

Compresses, sometimes referred to as fomentations, are pieces of clean cloth—often cotton, cheesecloth, or flannel—that have been soaked in an appropriate herbal infusion or decoction, wrung out, and then placed directly on an injury. They may be cool or hot, depending on the situation. They are often used for bruises, swellings, insect bites and stings, and sprains.

Compresses are easy enough to make while on the go, as long as you can make an herbal solution as described previously in the section on teas. Another method, easier when traveling, is to add several teaspoons of herbal tincture (described later in this chapter) to an equal amount of water, creating an instant infusion.

First, determine whether to use a hot or cold compress. A hot compress will increase or draw energy, whereas a cool compress will restrict it. (These guidelines also hold true for poultices and other forms of healing.) Next, decide which herbs to use. For example, imagine you wish to prepare a compress for someone who has sprained his or her ankle. This particular injury results in inflammation. Energetically, it's desirable to restrain the energy and decrease the inflammation. An ice pack would be a type of compress and probably the first item to use. Bags of frozen peas make excellent ice packs, because the small peas easily conform to the curves of the body. It's also possible to purchase ice packs specifically for traveling. After icing the sprain, you might want to apply a cool compress made from a St. John's wort and lobelia infusion.

To prepare this compress, first make an infusion of the herbs. Since the compress will be used externally, you'll want to make a strong infusion: Use three times the amount of herbs you'd use for an infusion taken internally. After straining the herbs, allow the infusion to cool. Soak a clean piece of cloth in the tea, remove it using tongs, and apply it to the sprain. You can wrap a dry cloth around this to keep it from dripping and making a mess.

If you're preparing a hot compress, you'll definitely need to use tongs to remove the cloth from the hot tea. Also, wearing gloves helps when folding the hot cloth. Before placing the compress on the body, make sure it's not too hot. Wrap the compress with a dry cloth to keep it warm.

Poultices

Poultices are moist herbs—either fresh or dried—applied to the skin. A poultice can also be made with clay or some other combination of liquid and solid material, as described in some of the examples below. They are used as treatments for bug bites or stings, skin eruptions, tumors or cysts, cuts and other wounds, boils, abscesses, and swollen glands. As a child, I spent my summers in Florida—primarily in a lake. Somehow, despite being in the water, I was constantly covered with mosquito bites, which I'd scratch fiercely until they bled and became infected. My mother would make bread-and-milk poultices—she'd dip a small piece of white bread in milk, slap it on the offending bite, and wrap it with gauze. By the next morning, the infection would be gone. I am a staunch believer in the poultice.

There are several categories of poultices to choose from, depending on the effect you're after. They are the heating or warming poultice, the soothing poultice, and the drawing poultice. A warming poultice is used to draw energy to a particular part of the body. The mustard poultice our grandmothers were so fond of is an excellent example. These were traditionally applied over the lungs to relieve congestion and bring healing warmth to these overtaxed organs. A soothing poultice is one used for irritated skin—rashes for example—or for injuries such as burns or sprains. The drawing poultice is used to pull out foreign matter, such as a splinter, that has become embedded in the skin. It can also be used for drawing out infectious material such as pus.

To make a poultice, mix your chosen material—clay or dried herbs—with a liquid to create a paste. Good moistening solutions include water, an herbal tea, apple cider, milk, and even essential oils, although these would probably be added to one of the liquids mentioned above. Soothing and warming poultices are usually made with a hot or warm solution. The resulting paste can be applied either directly to the skin or, more often, to gauze or a clean tea towel that has also been moistened and is then placed on the skin. As with compresses, wrap the poultice with a dry cloth; wool works best to keep the heat in. A hot-water bottle may be used on top of the dry cloth to further retain the heat.

Always use sterilized cloth, especially if it is to be placed on broken skin. This may be more difficult while you're on the road, so buy packaged, sterilized gauze or sterilize the cloth yourself by boiling it in water for 20 minutes. Use tongs to remove the cloth from the boiling water. Another rule of thumb is to use a poultice only once—it should never be reused. From a purely energetic standpoint, I don't think it would be wise to reuse a poultice that has drawn out congested energy. From a pathological viewpoint, just as you would not reuse a bandage that might contain infection, you would not want to use a poultice a second time. And finally, do use cloth for a poultice when you plan to place it over a hairy or sensitive area. When the herbs have dried, they're sometimes difficult to remove if you placed them directly on the skin. You wouldn't want to have to scrub an already irritated or painful area.

OILS AND SALVES

These are probably my favorite herbal support tools. They have numerous applications, feel good, store and travel well, and they work! Both are quite easily prepared on your own prior to traveling.

Herbal Oils

Herbal oils can be made from any fixed oil, such as sweet almond, grapeseed, peanut, or avocado, but many herbalists agree that the best oil, especially if it's to be used in a salve, is olive oil. This is so for several reasons.

First, olive oil is more stable and tends to keep longer than other oils. Never use any rancid oil when making herbal products. Much research has been done on the effects of rancidity in oil on human health. Rancidity is caused by the oxidation of fats. You should be able to tell if an oil has gone bad by smelling it. It will have the familiar metallic odor of stale potato chips—chips whose fat has become rancid. In fat, oxidation results in highly reactive molecules that damage components of human cells—in particular, a cell's DNA. There is evidence that this may lead to cancer, faster aging through tissue degeneration, and inflammatory and immune-system-related diseases.

A second reason to use olive oil is that it's nutritive in and of itself. Finally, it's made from the fruit of peace, the olive, and the olive branch has been used throughout history to symbolize peace. I couldn't think of a better oil to put on my skin when I wanted to calm it.

There are several methods for making herbal oils. Two easy ones are the indirect- and the direct-heat methods.

Indirect-Heat Method

To make herbal oil using the indirect-heat method, fill a clean jar two-thirds full with herbs, being careful not to pack them down. Then fill the jar all the way to the top with one of the fixed oils mentioned above. Cover the jar with a lid. You can either place the jar in a warm place in your house that's out of direct sunlight—the top of the refrigerator is perfect as long as it's not near a sunny window—or put the jar in a brown paper bag and let it sit outside in the sun. Let the jar remain for three to four days to infuse. (Some herbs, such as St. John's wort, take longer to infuse.) At this point you can strain the herbs from the oil. I find that this easiest to do by lining a large sieve with a clean cotton cloth—cheesecloth works well, as do remnants of old, clean sheets. Place the lined sieve over a bowl, which will catch the herbal oil. Pour the oil and herbs from the jar into the sieve and let it drain. (If you use a cloth with a tighter weave, such as a piece of sheeting, it will take longer to drain.) Once most of the oil is in the bowl, you can squeeze out the remainder by wringing the cloth and herbs over the sieve. Be sure to have washed your hands prior to doing this. The oil is now ready to be bottled and used.

Fresh herbs make wonderful oils. In fact, there are some oils that can be made only with fresh herbs—St. John's wort oil is one of them. These are a little trickier because of the water contained in the fresh plant material. There is an increased chance—a pretty good one, actually—that the water will separate from the plant as it infuses in the oil, becoming a breeding ground for mold. Mold in your oil can render it useless. One way to overcome this problem is to let the herb "dry-wilt" before using it. To dry-wilt means to let the herb dry partially. It should not be so dry that it crackles; nor should it be totally fresh. Somewhere in between, the dry-wilted plant will appear limp and shriveled. If you use fresh herbs in your oil, check the jar every day and wipe out any moisture from around the mouth of jar and the lid.

Another method I have used successfully with fresh herb material is to cover the jar with a paper towel, held in place with a rubber band. Daily stir the mixture slowly with a chopstick, letting air bubbles rise to the surface. Make sure to replace the paper towel, because it not only keeps debris out of the oil but also lets water evaporate as the oil is warmed slowly. It would be prudent to check the mouth of the jar for signs of water, just as you would with the dry-wilt process.

Direct-Heat Method

This is a quicker way to make herbal oil than the indirect-heat process. Its only drawbacks are that with direct heat, the medicinal properties of the plant may be diminished, and you might occasionally end up with burned plant material, rendering the oil useless. If you're careful, this shouldn't be a problem.

To use the direct-heat method, place the herbs in the top portion of a double boiler. Cover them with oil so that no plant material is sticking up beyond the surface of the oil, and cover the pot with a lid. After adding the appropriate amount of water to the bottom portion of the double boiler, place the container with the oil and herb mixture on top. Allow this to sit over direct heat on your stove for 45 minutes. Check the oil frequently to make sure that the oil is not so hot as to overheat or fry the herbs. You can stir and smell it occasionally during this time to help make sure that the temperature of the oil remains low. After 45 minutes, the oil and herbs are ready to be strained. Use the same process for straining as noted for the indirect method, above. Be sure to let the herbs and oil cool adequately before trying to squeeze out any remaining oil. I've burned myself more than once due to impatience. If you're using fresh herbs, don't try to wring the oil from the lining. Doing so might squeeze out remaining water from the herb, and this might lead to mold, as mentioned above.

A double boiler is not a requirement for the direct-heat method: You can also place both plant and oil directly into a saucepan and heat it. If you use this method, however, the heat must remain low and you must stir the mixture the entire time to ensure that the herb is not overcooked or fried.

Oil Choices

Which oil you choose to use in a preparation is based primarily upon the results you wish to obtain. Grapeseed oil is one of the lightest of oils and is used when making skin care products for those with oily skin. Avocado oil is rich and nourishing, and more appropriate for people with dry, flaky skin. Sweet almond oil makes an excellent base for massage oils; it's a medium-weight oil good for normal skin types. If you're making a medicinal salve, olive oil remains the best choice. One note of caution: an individual who is allergic to nuts may also respond poorly to an herbal oil or salve made from nut oils. It would be wise not to use nut oils at all in such cases.

Salves and Balms

Salves are one of my favorite remedies to make. A salve, or balm (as it is also called), offers endless ways to use herbs. There is something magical and ultimately healing about a salve. Perhaps they conjure up memories of childhood when mothers rubbed vapor balm onto congested chests and whispered healing words. I love them because they remind me of the little jars filled with strong-smelling unguents that my grandfather had in his medicine chest. And making one is analogous to canning the vegetable garden's bounty: All the medicinal properties of the herbs are locked away for a time of need. The same can be said for tinctures, but more about that in the next section.

Salves are tremendously easy to prepare. They're primarily made of herb-infused oils and beeswax, but other things can be added to increase the effectiveness of the resulting balm. Optional ingredients include vitamin E oil, honey, PABA, grapefruit seed extract, natural coloring, and essential oils. Shatoiya de la Tour, an excellent herbalist, teacher, and dear friend, suggests using rosemary, lavender, or thyme as part of the base oil blend for salves: Thyme contains thymol, which acts as a bacterial retardant, and rosemary and lavender act as preservatives.

To make a salve, add small pieces of beeswax to warm oil and allow them to melt slowly. I generally put my herbal oil in the top of a double boiler, warm it gently, then add my premeasured grated beeswax. Another way is to melt beeswax in an old heat-resistant measuring cup—just stick it in a warm oven with a tray underneath to catch any drips—then add the correct amount to the warmed oil. You can use the measurement markers on the side of the measuring cup to guide you. Make sure that the oil is warm before you add the beeswax. If it isn't, the hot, melted beeswax will solidify in the oil and create a congealed mess. This method is probably a little more riskier than the first, since it means having an open container of wax in the oven. Also, you won't be able to use the measuring cup for anything else once you've melted beeswax in it.

A general guideline for the oil-to-beeswax ratio is $2\frac{1}{2}$ cups of oil to 2 ounces of beeswax. This is not an exact science, however, and you'll need to test the consistency of your salve before pouring it into jars. To test the consistency, put a small amount of the oil-and-beeswax mixture in a spoon and place this in the freezer for about a minute to solidify. If the result is too firm, add more oil (warmed). If it's too soft, add more beeswax, but only a little at a time—it goes a long way.

Salves are excellent for aching muscles, congested chests, cuts, abrasions—essentially any external location to which you want to deliver the healing properties of herbs. One note of waring: Be careful if you're suffering from poison oak, ivy, or sumac. When the blisters are first forming, using an oil-based preparation might spread the reaction. You can use salves later, after the skin has dried up and is crusty and scabby. See the section on poison oak, ivy, and sumac for more treatment options.

TINCTURES AND LINIMENTS

Tinctures and liniments are made in exactly the same way. The only difference is that tinctures are used internally, whereas liniments are always used externally.

Tinctures

Tinctures, also called extracts, are among the easiest herbal remedies to take. They're more convenient than infusions—you can carry a 1-ounce bottle of tincture anywhere—and you don't have to boil water or wait. Tinctures also deliver the herbal constituents to the bloodstream faster. In addition, while dried herbs lose their potency fairly quickly (often within a year, depending on harvesting and storage conditions), tinctures retain their effectiveness for five years or longer. Rosemary Gladstar says she has known tinctures to retain their strength for more than twenty years.

This brings me to the topic of herbal solvents—the base for the extract, also referred to as the menstruum. Don't let the word *solvent* throw you off, even if it does sound like something you'd use to clean a corroded battery. A solvent is nothing more than the liquid in which the herbal constituents are dissolved. There are three different solvents, or menstruums, that can be used effectively when making tinctures: alcohol, glycerin, and vinegar. Each has its own set of advantages and disadvantages. In addition, certain herbal constituents can be rendered only in a particular menstruum. For instance, there are many alkaloids that wouldn't dissolve in either vinegar or glycerin.

Alcohol is the most commonly used solvent for herbal extracts. This is so for several reasons. First, alcohol will dissolve more plant constituents than either vinegar or glycerin. Since it's mixed with water, those constituents soluble in water only will also be included. Second, there's much more research and information available on what plant constituents dissolve in alcohol and how high a ratio of alcohol to water is required to render the constituents soluble. There is a downside, however— the alcohol makes a tincture inappropriate for recovering alcoholics. Parents may also be concerned about using an alcohol-based tincture for their children. To do so safely, place the drops into a glass of hot water. Most of the alcohol will dissipate with the heat. If alcohol is still a concern, however, parents can use glycerites—glycerin-based extracts—instead.

Both vinegar and glycerin are nutritive, so while they may not be as effective at dissolving plant constituents as alcohol, they have the extra benefit of supporting health in their own right. Glycerin is a chemical constituent found in oils, and may be either plant or animal derived. I prefer to use vegetable glycerin, which is available through mail order (see appendix B, Resources, at the end of this book) or at most health food stores. Glycerin makes an excellent extract for children. It's soothing and, because of its sweet taste, helps mask some of the more bitter flavors of herbs. I will say, however, that my son now enjoys the taste of echinacea so much that he refuses the glycerite version. Keep your glycerites refrigerated, if possible, for a longer shelf life.

Extracts made with vinegar can, of course, be used as a food. I can't think of a better way to take my medicine than in my daily salad. It sure is a great way to help better your family's health—they need never know! Just don't tell the kids how healthy it is for them. Apple cider vinegar is one of the oldest solvents used to extract herbal properties. It contains some minerals and is relatively acidic, which helps with the digestive process. While glycerites don't keep as long as alcohol-based tinctures, vinegar extracts can keep for several years or more. Let your nose be your guide. If it smells sour or begins to ferment and bubble, don't use it.

Making Tinctures

Making a tincture is similar to making an herbal oil. Both are processes that render herbal properties soluble in a menstruum. While there are more complex methods for making an alcohol-based tincture, such as the cold-percolation and standardized methods, the easiest is the simplers method. I have used this technique for years and found all my extracts to be just as effective as those available in stores—at a much lower cost. There are a number of pros and cons about which method to use and how to standardize, but that subject is best left to another book.

The simplers method is called such because it was the process used and passed down by simplers. These were (and are) folks who saw the connection between nature and health and chose to make their healing preparations in a simple way—often with only one herb.

A Simpler's Alcohol Tincture

1. Grind herbs. Use either a mortar and pestle or a small coffee grinder (be sure not to use this for your coffee as well!). The herbs don't have to be powdered, but you do want to break them up a bit to provide more surface area for the menstruum to work with.

2. Fill a clean, glass jar about halfway with the chosen plant material.

3. Pour alcohol over the herbs until the alcohol meets the top of the rim. Cover the jar with waxed paper and then screw the lid on tight. The waxed paper prevents leakage and allows easy removal of the lid later.

4. Shake the macerating herbs once a day to help the extraction process.

5. Let the herbs macerate for at least two weeks before straining. If you can wait six weeks, you'll have a stronger tincture.

6. When you're ready to strain the tincture from the herbs, place a clean cloth—cotton sheeting or cheesecloth—in a

sieve resting over a nonaluminum bowl. Slowly pour the tincture and herbs into the cloth and let it drain. To get as much of the tincture as possible, you'll need to squeeze the herbs inside the cloth. Strong hands are made from such work! It's also possible to buy an herb press, although for home use this probably isn't necessary.

7. Bottle the resulting tincture, preferably in brown bottles. Make sure to label these. You'd be surprised how many of us think we'll remember later what's in the jar and then are unable to do so. Include what herbs were used, when the extract was made, what alcohol was used, and what the tincture should be used for and how often.

I like to think thoughts such as "help and heal" while I'm shaking my jars, but this may be more than some people feel comfortable with. Store your tinctures in a cool, dark place, but one where you'll see them on a daily basis to remind you to shake them.

A word about what kind of alcohol to use: Vodka, brandy, and rum are all fine; it really is a matter of personal preference and taste. Some plant constituents require a higher percentage of alcohol to be dissolved. A higher proof means a larger ratio of alcohol to water. For example, 80-proof vodka indicates 40 percent alcohol and 60 percent water, while 100-proof means 50 percent of each. I generally use 80-proof vodka because it's easiest for me to obtain and I find that it works reasonably well.

If you're using fresh herbs in your tincture, rather than grinding them, bruise them a little. You don't have to worry about mold (as you do with an herbal oil), because the alcohol keeps bacteria and molds from growing.

Vinegar tinctures are made in the same manner as alcohol tinctures. Glycerites (glycerin tinctures) are only a little different.

Glycerin Tincture

1. Follow steps 1 and 2 for an alcohol tincture as described earlier in this section.

2. Using a mixture of half glycerin and half distilled water, fill the jar containing the herbs to the top. Cover the jar with waxed paper and then screw the lid on tight

3. The remaining steps are the same as for the alcohol tincture.

4. Although vegetable glycerin is a preservative, you should store your glycerites in the refrigerator to prolong their shelf life. They should keep for at least a year.

Liniments

A liniment is always used externally and is often made with rubbing alcohol as the menstruum. Liniments are made in the same manner as are alcohol tinctures. They're often used to bring deep, penetrating relief to aching muscles, as well as to dry up weepy skin conditions such as dermatitis resulting from exposure to poison oak, ivy, or sumac.

One of the most famous liniments is Dr. Kloss's Liniment, made with goldenseal, myrrh, and cayenne. In addition to drying up oozing dermatitis, Dr. Kloss's Liniment is an excellent disinfectant for cuts and wounds. Because it's made with rubbing alcohol, it should be diluted prior to use. Please see the section on cuts, scrapes, and abrasions for more information on this liniment, or read Dr. Kloss's book *Back to Eden* for the exact recipe.

CAPSULES AND SYRUPS

While capsules and syrups are nothing like each other in terms of preparation, they are two of the more familiar methods of ingesting "medicine." This often increases their chance of use. Both are easy to prepare and to take.

Capsules

I often wonder what *exactly* is in the herbal capsules I purchase already prepared at the pharmacy or health food store. There's no sure way to tell how long the herbs have been sitting on the shelf, how long they were at the manufacturer's facilities, and how much time elapsed before they were delivered to the manufacturer. If you have the patience to grow, dry, and encapsulate your own herbs, you'll always be assured of their freshness and viability. I must admit that I purchase most of my herbs, having only a small garden, but I'm comfortable with my sources and the freshness of the plant material.

You can purchase empty capsules at most health food stores and through the mail. Vegetable-based capsules are more common these days than they used to be, and are more ecologically sound than the gelatin capsules manufactured from horse hooves. They come in a variety of sizes, of which 0 and 00 are the most common. I generally use size 00—any bigger and they can be difficult to swallow; any smaller and they become cumbersome to fill. When

I first started capping my own herbs, I used the old-fashioned method, which works just fine except for being extremely tedious. There are now little gadgets you can buy that let you prepare fifty capsules at a time. They are inexpensive and well worth it. See appendix B to locate a source.

One trick to producing good capsules is to start with well-ground herbs. Some of the more resinous or hard plant parts, such as roots and bark, are very difficult to grind well in a coffee grinder. In these cases you should purchase your herbs preground. Leaves and aerial parts will grind to a powder with little effort.

◆

OLD-FASHIONED METHOD FOR CAPSULES

1. Grind herbs and mix them well in a bowl.

2. Take apart capsules, making sure to retain all the tops.

3. Using the two halves of a capsule, scoop up the powdered herb and push the ends together to form a well-filled capsule.

It takes a little practice to get the right amount of herb and to be able to close the capsule, but it isn't difficult. In many cases a treatment will call for 2 capsules three times a day. It helps to make a lot of capsules, at least 50 at a time, so you don't have to sit down and do this every day—especially if you aren't feeling well. Store your capsules in a jar with a tight-fitting lid to keep moisture from softening them. Remember to label the jar with the date, ingredients, and what they're used for.

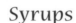

Syrups

I prefer syrups for administering herbal preparations to small children. They're especially useful when a sore throat or cough is present, because the syrup helps coat the inflamed tissues. Syrups are fun to make and, because they contain honey and/or glycerin, their taste is often preferable to some of the more bitter teas. Glycerin is a nutritive and a natural preservative. Honey has healing properties of its own and is excellent at cutting through mucus to deliver the herb's therapeutic properties.

SYRUP PREPARATION

1. Using 1quart of water to approximately 2 ounces of herb, prepare an infusion or decoction of the required herbs.

2. Slowly simmer the tea until the liquid has been reduced by half.

3. Strain the herbs from the tea.

4. While the tea is still warm, add 2 ounces of honey and/or glycerin and stir until dissolved.

5. Optional: Add $\frac{1}{4}$ cup of brandy as an additional preservative.

6. Bottle, label, and store in the refrigerator. The syrup will keep for about one month.

2
AROMATHERAPY
◆

ESSENTIAL OILS ARE THE SUBSTANCE OF AROMA-
therapy, which is the use of essential oils to bring about positive
change in health and well-being. Aromatherapy is a study unto
itself, and this book makes no attempt to discuss it thoroughly as a
healing art. There are a number of wonderful books published on
the subject, many of which are noted in the bibliography. In
general, essential oils are used in very small amounts, which means
small bottles that are easy to carry when you're traveling. More
important, they're often excellent remedies for the kinds of
ailments you might experience while on a journey.

An important constituent of many herbs is their volatile oils.
These oils are what give many plants their characteristic scent,
such as the thymol in thyme. Volatile oils are collected from the
plant most often through distillation. Essential oils are called such
because they are truly the essence of the plant. I believe that
essential oils are a combination of the lifeblood of the plant and
a bit of its spirit, as well.

Production of an essential oil requires an enormous amount of plant material. The numbers are, in fact, staggering and explain the often high costs associated with pure essential oils, which are sold as true commodities. The amount of essential oil you can obtain from a plant depends on a number of factors, an important one being the percentage of volatile oil in the plant. This differs with each species. An example is rosemary, which contains a relatively high percentage of volatile oils. It requires approximately 500 pounds of rosemary plants to yield 2 pounds of essential oil. In comparison, rose petals are relatively low in volatile oils. Up to 2,000 pounds of rose petals are required to produce 1 pound of pure rose essential oil.

Most, if not all, essential oils have antibacterial and antiseptic properties due to their chemical components, notably terpenes, phenols, alcohols, and aldehydes. This makes them an excellent component in external first-aid remedies. Note the word *external*. While it's a fact that essential oils can be used internally with relative safety, do not attempt this unless you're under the care of a trained and trusted aromatherapist. Many essential oils would be toxic if used internally, so to do so safely requires years of study. I have heard several tragic stories about the consequences—death in some cases—and believe that internal use of essential oils is best left to the practitioner.

Clearly, essential oils are powerful substances. Even external use requires dilution in most cases. Lavender essential oil is one of the few that can be used neat—that is, applied directly to the skin without prior dilution. Generally, essential oils are diluted in a carrier oil or water, which may then be applied in the form of massage oil, bath oil, salve, soap, cream, wash, or spray.

There are, in my opinion, four required essential oils for

every travel first-aid kit. With these four, you can alleviate a number of problems and often find relief. They are lavender, peppermint, tea tree, and eucalyptus. I always carry both lavender and peppermint essential oils in my purse, and I use them all the time. Air sickness and other forms of nausea can frequently be eased by sniffing peppermint oil.

Recently, my husband and I were flying home after attending a business conference. Our plane was attempting to land at night during a vicious rainstorm in 30-mph winds. Needless to say, folks were overwhelmed by the turbulence and were randomly becoming sick. I noticed my husband was pale and waxy looking, sure signs of nausea. I handed him my bottle of peppermint essential oil and by taking frequent sniffs of the aroma, he was able to overcome his queasiness.

Essential oils for specific problems are noted and considered as part of most ailments in chapter 6. I leave you with one of my favorite essential oil recipes, an antiseptic and freshening spray. It contains lavender and thyme oils, both of which are antiseptic and specific to lung infections. I use it in the bathroom as a room freshener—I prefer it to the natural ones on the market—and to spray in a sickroom. You might like to use it in your hotel room.

Room-Freshening Spray

1. Fill a 2-ounce glass spray bottle with distilled water.
2. Add to it 7 drops of lavender oil and 4 drops of thyme oil.
3. Replace the spray top and spray!

3
HOMEOPATHY

ALTHOUGH PRACTICED WIDELY IN EUROPE AND India and used by the British royals, homeopathy has only recently gained popularity in the United States. Developed in the early 1800s by Samuel Hahnemann, a German physician, homeopathy is based on the principle of "like cures like" and works by stimulating the body's ability to heal itself. Homeopathic remedies are made from the same animal, mineral, and plant materials that, if given to an individual, would bring about the same set of symptoms the homeopathic dose is meant to cure. A homeopathic dose is prepared by diluting the material with water or alcohol repeatedly. Different strengths can be created: The more dilute a remedy, the stronger its action. Many of the substances used to create a homeopathic remedy would be toxic in their normal form. Belladonna is one example.

Classic homeopathy dictates that for the modality to work successfully, it is necessary to match an individual's symptoms to the appropriate remedy. There are more than one thousand individual remedies, so it can be quite painstaking to do so. Generally speaking, this sort of diagnosis is best left in the hands of a trained homeopath. There are a number of single remedies available, however, that have a specific use for the general population and can be employed easily and readily. An example is arnica, which is used for muscle and joint pain resulting from injury, such as a sprain, bruise, or pulled muscle. Additionally, there are available combinations of remedies, often called complexes, which address general complaints such as flu or allergies. Oscillococcinum is a good example of a complex used to treat flu (see the section on colds and flu). These complexes generally contain around six to eight different remedies, that treat specific symptoms individually but, when combined, provide a shotgunlike approach to a universal complaint.

Homeopathic remedies should be taken 30 minutes before or after ingesting anything except water. Most come in the form of a small tablet or minute pill. These are placed under the tongue and allowed to dissolve slowly in the mouth. A general rule of thumb is not to touch the pill(s) before putting them in your mouth. Some remedies come in special dispensers that allow you to measure out three to five pills and drop them into your mouth without having to touch them with your fingers. In other cases you can tap a few pills in the bottle's lid and then toss them into your mouth. Try not to ingest mint when using homeopathic products. Traditional thought says that constituents in mint will interfere with the homeopathic remedy's effectiveness (although I know a number of practitioners who dispute this idea). Homeopathic remedies are generally considered safe, even for infants, although caution should always be used if you're making your own diagnosis. For more information on homeopathy, see appendix B, Resources.

4
FLOWER ESSENCES

❖

LIKE AROMATHERAPY, FLOWER ESSENCES ARE A
separate subject—and not one that I can do justice to in this small
book. However, since every natural first-aid kit should contain
a bottle of Rescue Remedy, one of the original flower essences
intuited by Dr. Edward Bach, it seems worthwhile to offer an
introduction to the subject.

Dr. Edward Bach was a British physician who obtained his
medical degree at Cambridge in the early 1900s. He practiced in
London, England, working at the labs of the Royal London
Homeopathic Hospital. Unlike many physicians of the time (and
perhaps currently), Dr. Bach was more interested in the patient
than the disease. During his research at the Royal London
Homeopathic Hospital, he discovered that a particular homeopathic remedy could be given to an individual with good results
based not on physical symptoms, but rather on the person's
emotions at the time. This confirmed for him what he already
suspected: that physical disease results from an imbalance in a
person's mental attitude.

Growing disillusioned with medicine as it was performed in his day, he gave up his London practice and moved to Wales, his family home. He felt, intuitively, that he would be led to new homeopathic remedies in nature, walking the verdant hills and valleys of his homeland. One story says that when Dr. Bach left London, he packed two similar bags—one containing his medical instruments and the other, shoes to be given away. However, upon arriving in Wales, he realized that the bag he'd left for charity contained not his shoes, but rather his medical instruments. Undaunted, Dr. Bach felt this to be a sign confirming that he would indeed find the remedies he was looking for in nature. Certainly he would need the shoes for all the walking he'd be doing!

The manner in which Dr. Bach discovered his thirty-eight remedies is interesting, if not bordering on the fantastic. On occasion he was afflicted with a particular negative mental state, often accompanied by physical symptoms. This prompted him to look for a remedy. Traveling the countryside, he would find a flower that would quickly relieve his symptoms and renew his sense of peace and wellness. This experience, then, was the *proving*—a homeopathic term indicating proof that an extremely minute dosage of a particular substance would relieve the symptoms it would also bring on if taken in much larger amounts.

The actual flower essences are produced in a precise process that involves capturing the essence of the flower in pure springwater at a particular time of day. The essences themselves work to restore a specific "positive mental state" associated with the flower, and will also relieve physical symptoms that might also be present.

The most famous of Dr. Bach's flower essences, Rescue Remedy, is actually a composite of five specific essences:

1. Cherry Plum, for loss of emotional control
2. Clematis, for the feeling you have prior to fainting
3. Impatiens, for when you're agitated and cannot relax
4. Rock Rose, for intense panic and fear
5. Star of Bethlehem, for shock

It's easy to see why this particular remedy is so useful for first aid.

If you have no experience with homeopathy or vibrational medicine, it might be difficult to accept that a flower essence has any effect at all—except perhaps as a placebo. But I have seen Bach flower therapy work so well on my cats, which have neither the intellect nor the predilection to understand placebo effect, that I must believe in its effectiveness.

Rescue Remedy may be given internally, 2 to 4 drops under the tongue, or can be used externally directly on the skin. Because it does contain brandy, recovering alcoholics should apply it externally. It should be used at any time when you're suffering from shock, have been wounded, or must deal with others who are injured. A car accident would be one such time. I use it on my cats, rubbing a few drops on the backside of their ears, prior to visiting the vet. My son gets a dose before and after visits to the dentist. His stepmother and I used it on him during a recent surgery—he seemed to recover much more quickly and experienced less anesthetic-related vomiting than with prior surgeries. Rescue Remedy can also be added to healing salves, teas, compresses, poultices, and sprays (spritzers). Shatoiya de la

Tour always adds a few drops to the water when she's seeding and transplanting seedlings. You may also purchase Rescue Remedy cream, which would also be a worthwhile addition to the first-aid kit.

While Bach flower essences are the originals, there are many new flower essences being made, both in this country and elsewhere. In my opinion they work equally well and are excellent additions to the healing repertoire. For more information about Rescue Remedy, specific flower essences, or how they are made, see appendix B.

5

MAKING A TRAVELER'S

◆

MEDICINE KIT

MAKING YOUR OWN FIRST-AID KIT IS AN ADVEN-
ture. It requires planning and ingenuity. It may remind you of
childhood games—scavenger hunts come to mind. Don't expect
it to be an inexpensive proposition, and don't expect to complete
it in a day—unless you're a terrific planner.

You'll likely want more than one first-aid kit, depending on
its intended use. I have a big one for home, a little one for
backpacking, and a slightly larger one for travel by air, boat, or
car. What you put in your kits is largely up to you and will depend
upon your and your family's needs. It will also depend upon
where you're traveling. It's a highly individual endeavor. For
instance, I have a bottle of Herb Pharm's Propolis/Echinacea
Spray in all my kits, because my throat seems to be the first place
to show signs of distress when I'm coming down with
something—and this spray is great for sore throats. In addition,
it's one of those items that do double duty: I have used it with

good results as a spray for cuts, abrasions, and bug bites. On the other hand, someone in your family might have a propensity for athlete's foot. In this case, you'd probably want to include a remedy in your travel kit. Since your kit is an individual creation and the overall goal is to include what you know works for you, please don't stress about throwing in some over-the-counter remedy, even if it is synthetic. I have Sudafed in my kits because it's about the only thing that works effectively for me if I'm traveling by air and become congested. In my opinion it's better to take the "dreaded" pill than to deal with a deep, full-blown ear infection two days later due to my body's inability to deal with air-pressure changes. This book is about natural remedies, but it's also about flexibility.

CARRYING IT ALL

What you use to carry all your healing goodies is, again, a matter of personal choice. I've seen all kinds of containers. The most impressive one I ever saw was Shatoiya de la Tour's—an enormous fishing tackle box. It has dozens of little plastic drawers and a pop-out kit the size of a lunch box that you can reach for quickly in a case of emergency. A box that size would not be your first choice on a Caribbean cruise, but I had to mention it here because of its "granddaddy" status. Other (less ambitious) containers that make useful kits include small baskets with lids, quilted makeup bags, tool kits, and small fishing tackle boxes. If you know someone good with a sewing machine, you might even consider commissioning a first-aid kit. I'd love to have one made out of quilted fabric with little pockets and elastic loops to hold tincture bottles in place. If designed well, it could easily roll up and store snugly in your carry-on. Still, the bottom line is that what you use to carry your first-aid supplies is totally up to you.

Remedies that might melt or containers that could leak or spill should be individually placed in plastic bags to prevent seepage onto your clothes or elsewhere in your travel bags. Save empty film canisters for storing small items such as pills or sewing items. One note of warning: Do not store loose dried herbs in film canisters for travel. These canisters used to be the number one choice for carrying small, personal-use amounts of marijuana back in the 1960s and 1970s. Any loose dried plant that is green, brown, or somewhere in between is going to look suspicious to most customs officials, especially if it's in a film canister. You definitely do not want to spend your arrival day in customs sorting out what could become quite nasty, depending on your destination. See Navigating Customs later in this chapter for more information.

Essential oils must be stored in glass vials or bottles. The constituents in essential oils will eat right through a plastic container, as well as the rubber bulb at the end of a glass dropper. When buying essential oils for travel, always get them with a solid screw top. Some come with dispensers built into the bottles but, if not, buy individual glass droppers (one for each bottle) and store them separately. Tincture bottles should either be stored in individual compartments (that's why tackle kits are so great) or placed in plastic bags. The 1-ounce size is obviously smaller and would pack more easily, but you might consider a larger bottle for something like echinacea that the whole family will use.

Make sure all your remedies are labeled. It's so tempting, especially if you're packing at the last minute, to think you'll remember what it is that you poured into that brown tincture bottle. Believe me, noses aren't infallible, and even lavender essential oil can smell like rosemary essential oil if you have no context—such as the bottle's position on your shelf. It's even more difficult to sort out what's what with tinctures, and nearly impossible with capsules. I am embarrassed to admit that I've thrown out my share of capsules simply because I couldn't remember what I put in them and I hadn't taken the time to label the jar. Obviously, labeling isn't necessary if you're buying premade remedies at your local health food store—unless, of course, you repackage them. Labels should list the name of the preparation and/or contents, what it's used for, whether it should be taken internally or externally (remember that others might use your kit) what the dosage is, and the date.

To help reduce repackaging, take advantage of promotional and trial-sized items. When I worked at an alternative "pharmacy" in Palo Alto, we had a fairly large display area of small trial- or travel-sized preparations. Among other things, you could get ¼-ounce tins of Tiger Balm and small plastic tubes of calendula ointment or aloe vera gel. Many of our vendors supplied us with promotional items that we gave away to customers at the checkout stand. So be on the lookout when shopping—you never know what you might find.

PLANNING YOUR KIT

The idea is simple: You should put as much time and effort into packing your first-aid kit—maybe more—as you would into packing the rest of your personal belongings. The size and number of your kits and what you put in them depend entirely upon your destination, your mode of travel, the length of your trip, the activities you plan to engage in, and who's going along. You might want to customize your kits for each trip, but at least your smallest everyday kit will usually remain pretty much the same. Remember to go through your kits at least once a year to replace used items and discard old ones.

The following is a list of questions to help you begin thinking of what you might want to put in your travel kit(s). If you are an experienced traveler, some of the items may seem obvious, but it pays to think about all the elements of your kit so you can choose remedies that will do double or triple duty. Is there a headache remedy that will also relieve insomnia, soothe sunburn, and (if you are a woman) ease menstrual cramps? Anything you can do to make your kit lighter while keeping it as complete as possible will make for a more pleasant trip. I like the idea of having two different kits—a larger one that goes in my luggage and a smaller one for my purse or carry-on. If you're backpacking, you'll most likely have room for only a small kit, and you'll probably want to keep everything together in one place.

1. **What is the length of your trip?** The longer your trip, the greater the likelihood that you'll need a wider variety of remedies.

2. **What's your destination?** You might decide not to take along items that you know can be gotten easily at your travel destination. For example, if you're going to see family, you probably wouldn't bother to take along an Ace bandage; but you'd likely take one if you're going backpacking. Also, think about the water: You might want to pack along tablets for water purification or Citricidal (an effective antiparasitic synthesized from grapefruit seeds and pulp). If you're going

someplace sunny, take aloe vera gel for possible sunburn treatment. And remember to think about what might look suspicious to customs agents. Don't take along items that might get you into trouble.

3. **Does your kit need to be waterproof?** Most standard business trips won't require a waterproof first-aid kit, but if your vacation consists of kayaking, rafting, or sailing, you'll want your remedies to be watertight.

4. **Who's going on this trip?** Take along items you think might be needed by any other members of your family traveling with you. If you have children, definitely take along a thermometer or temperature strips.

5. **What will you be doing on this trip?** Think about the activities you'll be engaging in and what might happen as a result. It sounds like planning for the worst, but really it's just being prepared. If you're traveling for business, stress is likely the most serious thing you'll suffer, so make sure to pack kava tincture or capsules and some lavender essential oil. If you'll be walking a lot, be sure to carry along some adhesive bandages and/or moleskin.

6. **For women:** Are you expecting your menstrual period, and if so are there any special remedies you might want along? If you're prone to cramps, you might consider taking along a remedy specifically for them.

NAVIGATING CUSTOMS

If you're traveling out of the country, you'll deal with customs. Depending on your destination, the experience could be as easy as choosing the "green" lane and walking through to the other side. In other countries, agents will stop everyone and go through their belongings as a matter of course. One year, my sister and I were traveling home to Iran for Christmas. We rather stupidly had wrapped all of our Christmas presents before packing them. To this day, I can't imagine what we were thinking. We had grown up in the Middle East, were well acquainted with customs procedures in that area of the world, and knew we had an excellent chance of being searched. Anyway, the woman going through our baggage tore the paper from each gift, examined the contents, threw the whole mess back in our bags and sent us on our way. It was an experience in violation and one that imparted a good lesson: be careful what you take with you and how you package it.

I haven't the knowledge to tell you what you can't take with you to each and every country. For one thing, the rules change more often than you'd imagine. While travel agencies might help, your best bet is to inquire at the embassies or consulates for the countries you plan to visit. Another idea is to call your health care practitioner and find out what advice he or she gives patients who travel. In general, though, it's wise to stay away from loose dried herbs. You'll probably be okay if they're in capsules, store bought, and labeled. I think I'd feel fine taking tea bags with me, especially if they were individually packaged in sealed envelopes. Don't take items that look suspicious.

Whenever I'm stopped and questioned about my personal belongings, I try to remain as cooperative as possible. This is not the time to take an attitude. Explaining sometimes helps, especially if language is not a barrier, but if officials want you to part with whatever is bothering them, let them do so.

SAMPLE KITS

To help you think about what you might want to include in your travel kits, here are a few sample kits. The first is my little kit that goes everywhere with me.

Sample Everyday Medicine Kit

¼-ounce bottle lavender essential oil

¼-ounce bottle peppermint essential oil

2–4 adhesive bandages

1 small bottle Rescue Remedy

4 decongestant tablets

1-ounce bottle echinacea tincture

arnica homeopathic tablets (30x strength)

¼-ounce tin all-purpose herbal salve

1-ounce bottle St. John's wort oil

1–2 individual packets antiseptic cleanser

2 throat lozenges

1 bottle Herb Pharm Echinacea/Propolis Spray

Sample Air Travel Kit

all the items listed under Sample Everyday Medicine Kit

1-ounce kava tincture

20 ginger capsules

witch hazel spritzer (and see the section on swollen feet or ankles).

Sample Backpacking First-Aid Kit

moleskin

Ace bandage

arnica homeopathic tablets (30x strength)

1 small bottle St. John's wort oil

¼-ounce bottle lavender essential oil

¼-ounce bottle tea tree essential oil

1 small container powdered yarrow or cayenne pepper

1 ounce shepherd's purse–yarrow tincture

1 ounce echinacea tincture

10–20 adhesive bandages (assorted sizes)

¼-ounce tin herbal antibiotic salve

water purifying tablets or Citricidal

2–4 antihistamine capsules

1 small jar green clay–lavender essential oil–echinacea–goldenseal-tincture paste

1 small bottle Dr. Kloss's Liniment

matches in a waterproof container

tweezers

Swiss Army knife

1–2 packs instant miso soup

Medium-Sized Travel Kit (packed in luggage)

If you're planning to also carry a small kit with you in your carry-on or purse, there's no need to duplicate the items in your medium-sized kit. Also, be sure to bring any prescription drugs that you take on a regular basis. Replacing these while traveling may be quite difficult.

- $1/4$-ounce bottles lavender essential oil, peppermint essential oil, German chamomile essential oil, tea tree essential oil, and eucalyptus essential oil
- 2-ounce bottle echinacea tincture
- 1-ounce bottle kava tincture
- 1-ounce bottle valerian tincture
- 1-ounce bottle pain and anti-inflammatory tincture
- 1-ounce bottle bitters tincture
- 1 small container cayenne powder
- 2–6 bags peppermint tea
- 2–6 bags chamomile tea
- $1/4$-ounce tin multipurpose herbal salve
- $1/4$-ounce tin Tiger Balm
- 1 small bottle St. John's wort oil
- 6 vials Oscillococcinum
- 1 bottle arnica homeopathic tablets (30x strength)

1 bottle Rescue Remedy

1 bottle melatonin

2–4 vials of Curing Pills (Chinese patent remedy)

1 small bottle ginger capsules

1 small tube aloe vera gel

1 small jar green clay–echinacea–goldenseal–lavender essential oil paste

1 small bottle activated charcoal

1 small bottle Herb Pharm Echinacea/Propolis Spray

2–10 decongestant tablets

2–4 antihistamine capsules

Scissors (small pair)

5–10 adhesive bandages (assorted sizes)

thermometer

tampons or pads

tweezers

Possible Items for Your Kit

The following is a long, but not exhaustive, list of items you might consider for your kits, especially those you keep at home or take car camping. Again, don't feel you have to include the same things I have—you know your family and self better than anyone else.

Tinctures

echinacea tincture

echinacea-goldenseal tincture

shepherd's purse–yarrow tincture (bleeding)

kava tincture

valerian tincture

cramp bark–valerian tincture (menstrual cramping)

pain and anti-inflammatory tincture

bitters tincture

horsetail–goldenrod–juniper–corn silk tincture
(urinary tract infections)

Dried Loose Herbs (for tea or bleeding)

cayenne

yarrow

peppermint

chamomile

fennel seeds

Salves

all-purpose herbal salve

calendula ointment or salve

herbal antibiotic salve

Tiger Balm

vapor balm (for congestion)

Herbal Oils

arnica oil (or gel)

St. John's wort oil

pain oil (arnica, St. John's wort, dandelion)

small bottle with plain vegetable oil
(for massage blends)

Essential Oils

lavender

peppermint

tea tree
eucalyptus
German chamomile
clary sage

Homeopathic Remedies and Flower Essences
Oscillococcinum
arnica homeopathic pills (30x strength)
Traumeel
Rescue Remedy
Rescue Remedy Cream

Supplements
vitamin C
acidophilus (nonrefrigerated type)
melatonin

Miscellaneous
Curing Pills (Chinese patent remedy)
Dr. Kloss's Liniment
Tiger Liniment
throat lozenges
Para-Gard
packets of instant miso soup
ginger capsules
cranberry capsules
cascara sagrada capsules
aloe vera gel
loose clay
green clay-echinacea-goldenseal-lavender paste (bug bites,
    poison oak)

activated charcoal
witch hazel spritzer
Herb Pharm Echinacea/Propolis Spray
decongestant
antihistamine

Supplies

gauze bandages
finger splint
tape
scissors (small pair)
pen and paper
matches
needle
adhesive bandages
thermometer
tampons or pads
Ace bandage
moleskin
flashlight
Citricidal
hot-water bottle
ice and heat bags
tweezers
Swiss Army knife

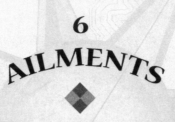

6
AILMENTS

◆

ABSCESSES

An abscess, or boil, is a painful, inflamed bump on the skin resulting from an accumulation of pus that has formed due to an infection somewhere in the body. Recurrent episodes of abscesses and boils generally point to a depressed immune system. A boil or abscess requires external treatment and may include lancing. Some abscesses, such as those of a dental nature, require professional help.

Bringing it To a Head

To bring a boil to a head, gather fresh plantain leaves and crush them with hot water. Plantain is a common weed that grows all over Europe, Asia, and the Americas. Both the broad-leaved *(Plantago major)* and the narrow-leaved *(P. lanceolata)* species may be used. If you aren't familiar with and easily able to identify the fresh plant, you can use dried plantain if you have it in your first-aid kit. Take the resulting herbal mash, cool it slightly so that it doesn't burn the skin, and apply it to the boil. A gauze bandage will help hold the plant material in place. This will soften the boil and draw the pus to the surface so that the infectious matter can be expelled. Apply tea tree oil several times a day to the area to clear up any infection. I have also used a clean washcloth soaked in a basin of hot water to which 10 drops of lavender essential oil have been added. Squeeze the hot water from the cloth and hold it to the abscess until it cools. Repeat several times. Be certain both the basin and your hands are clean.

Sometimes it's important to keep the abscess open so that it can drain. I have heard that it's possible to put a small "wick" made of clean gauze in the wound that will not only maintain an opening but will also draw out pus and other material. The gauze should be changed several times a day. This may not be possible with a small abscess.

A Typical Protocol for Clearing a Boil or Abscess

My son once got an abscess from an unclean earring, obtained while traveling, I might add. Several days later, when he returned home, he asked me to loosen the stud because it was "too tight." As it turned out, the earlobe was swollen and quite inflamed with infection. I used the following protocol to clear the abscess, with one exception: Instead of applying the recommended clay poultice, I used an antibiotic ointment, not knowing that this would close up the abscess. The earlobe appeared to be healed for several days, even weeks, and then festered and became swollen again. This occurred four times. On the fourth time, I did two things differently. First, I used the clay poultice rather than the antibiotic ointment and second, suspecting a systemic infection, I gave my son echinacea-goldenseal tincture. (See appendix A, Children's Dosages.) The abscess did not return.

1. Wash your hands with hot, soapy water. It would also be appropriate to use sterile gloves.

2. Apply a clean washcloth that has been soaked in very hot water to the abscess to bring it to a head.

3. Squeeze the wound gently to discharge any pus. One note of caution: Do not squeeze too hard, because the infection can be driven into surrounding tissues. I have also used a sterilized needle at the base of the boil to create a small opening rather than squeezing hard.

4. After gently removing as much pus as possible, use a disinfectant such as Dr. Kloss's Liniment on a clean cotton ball to clean the abscess. For more information on this liniment, please see the section on cuts, scrapes, and abrasions.

5. Apply a clay poultice to draw out any remaining infection. See the following on how to make a clay poultice.

◆

DRYING CLAY POULTICE

I learned how to make this from Rosemary Gladstar one wonderful summer in Vermont.

1. In a small jar (1 to 2 ounces), place enough green clay (any dry cosmetic clay can be substituted) to fill the jar halfway.

2. Add distilled water to moisten the clay somewhat, but not so much that it reaches the consistency of paste yet.

3. Add enough echinacea-goldenseal tincture to create a stiff paste.

4. Finally, add 10 to 20 drops of lavender essential oil and stir. Tea tree oil may be substituted for the lavender, because both have strong disinfectant properties.

ALLERGIES, HAY FEVER, AND HIVES

Hay fever is the name given to a specific allergy to airborne pollens from hay and grass. The medical term is *allergic rhinitis.* Symptoms can range from mild to severe and include a runny nose, watery eyes, sneezing, and a general feeling of malaise. While normally not critical, if the allergy is severe enough, hay fever can induce a form of asthma, which can be serious.

All allergies, whether hay fever or not, are an inflammatory response to toxins the body is unable to cope with. Normally and under optimum conditions, our livers are able to process most offending toxins. I say *optimum* because these days there are so many exogenic (environmental) toxins with which our bodies must deal, that even relatively healthy individuals have become susceptible to allergies. Our livers have become overburdened and more and more often I hear people say that they've recently developed allergies they hadn't had as children.

Since allergies involve both the liver and the body's in-flammatory response, it's useful to treat both areas when dealing with allergies. There are also specific remedies for hay fever and the hives, which often accompany food allergies.

Working the Liver

An excellent herb for the liver is milk thistle *(Silybum marianum)*. It's both a tonic and a regenerative. I recommend taking this herb on a regular basis while traveling, whether or not you show symptoms of allergy, simply due to the way that the stresses of traveling can affect the liver. The recommended dosage is 30 to 40 drops of the tincture in a small glass of warm water three times a day.

I also recommend taking some kind of bitters on a daily basis, either as food or in a tincture. Bitters can be either a bitter salad green such as dandelion leaves or wild chicory, or a tonic formula made from bitter herbs. They strengthen the immune and nervous system and have a beneficial effect on the digestive system. If you're traveling in the Mediterranean countries, bitters should be easy enough to come by in your diet alone. Many of the bitter salad greens we eschew (unfortunately) in this country are widely available in places such as Italy, Greece, France, and many of the Middle Eastern countries. A popular dish in Iran and other Middle Eastern countries is called *sabzi*. Many Middle Eastern cultures have their own version, and all are delicious. In general, sabzi contains a mixture of raw, bitter greens. These are eaten prior to the main portion of the meal, somewhat like an appetizer, and they have the same effect that all bitters do on the digestive system, which is to stimulate the production of digestive enzymes and bile, thus ensuring a well-digested meal. Try including some sort of bitter green in your daily diet while traveling. If greens are unavailable, you can take bitters as a tincture half an hour before meals. Most health food stores sell a bitters formula; Swedish Bitters is a well-known example. And if you forget to include it in your kit, many bars and taverns will be happy to sell you the occasional aperitif made with either Campari or Angostura Bitters.

The Inflammatory Response

Despite its well-deserved reputation as a mild, gentle herb, chamomile *(Matricaria recutita)* has an excellent anti-inflammatory action and can be used successfully as a natural antihistamine. It's often a favorite herb because it can be given safely, even to children, and has so many differing beneficial properties that it should be included in all herbal first-aid kits. One note of caution: I have occasionally heard that since chamomile is in the same botanical family (Compositae) as ragweed, a plant often associated with hay fever, it should not be used as a treatment for allergic rhinitis. This doesn't make sense to me. Many of the most popular herbs are in the Compositae family and are used successfully every day without allergic reactions. They include dandelion *(Taraxacum officinale),* echinacea *(Echinacea* spp.), calendula *(Calendula officinalis),* and many more. The reality is that allergies are highly individual in nature; a person could be allergic to any number of herbs. I have also heard that less reputable sources of chamomile may include "grasses" in the mix, which are themselves responsible for the allergic reaction. If you at all suspect that you might be allergic to chamomile, either don't use it at all or try it in a very small quantity—a couple of sips of tea—and see whether you have any reaction. Actually, this is good advice when trying out any new herb, especially if multiple allergies are a problem for you. Be sure to buy your herbs from trusted sources.

The easiest way to take chamomile is as a tea. It's very calming and has a pleasant fresh "yellow" taste. That sounds unusual, I know, but once you try it, if you haven't already, you'll understand. The standard dose is 2 teaspoons of dried herb to 1 cup of hot water. Let it steep for 5 to 10 minutes before drinking. I find that steeping it longer imparts an unpleasant metallic aftertaste, but I seem to be the only person I know who feels this way, so see what you think. Start with 2 cups a day.

Turmeric *(Curcuma longa),* the spice used in Indian cuisine, is also an excellent anti-inflammatory and does double duty as a liver protective. Taken alone, it has a rather strong taste, but it's not at all difficult to find Indian food all over Europe and Asia, so it should be easy (as well as fun) to get it through your diet.

Another natural anti-inflammatory is bromelain. This term refers to a group of enzymes, capable of digesting protein, that are present in the stems of pineapples. There is evidence, supported by double-blind research, that bromelain is helpful for individuals with sinusitis. Sinusitis, an inflammation of the sinus passages, is sometimes a result of reactions to airborne allergens. The general recommendation for taking bromelain supplements is 2,000 MCU (milk clotting units) three times a day.

Specific Remedies for Hay Fever

Up until a couple years ago I took Claritin, a common prescription pharmaceutical, for my year-round allergies. I had been on it or some sort of prescription antihistamine for approximately ten years. Wanting to try a natural approach, I visited my health care practitioner, Dr. Lois Johnson, who recommended a personalized tincture based on my constitution and particular complaints. It has worked very well. One of the herbs in my formula is eyebright *(Euphrasia officinalis)*. Eyebright has both anti-inflammatory and astringent actions and has long been known as a specific herb for many eye conditions, such as conjunctivitis, and for problems associated with the mucous membranes. In particular, it seems to work well for the itchy, watery eyes associated with hay fever. It combines well with other herbs and is found in many popular allergy formulas available at health food stores. If you have allergies, it would be well worth your time to try out one or more of these formulas prior to traveling. One caution: I recommend staying away from formulas containing ma huang *(Ephedra sinica),* commonly listed as ephedra. Although a traditional herbal antihistamine, ephedra is a powerfully stimulating botanical that should be used with caution, especially if you have high blood pressure. It should never be given to children. All herbs will have varying degrees of potency depending on the environmental conditions where they were grown and the methods used to harvest and store the plant material. Ephedra, in particular, seems to vary substantially, and it can be difficult to find the correct dosage.

My favorite herb for assuaging the symptoms of hay fever is the common nettle *(Urtica dioica)*. Yes, this is the same plant known as stinging nettle that's often responsible for painful welts and a stinging sensation if you inadvertently bump into it while hiking. I like to think of it as a strong "teacher," helping the wayward individual become more aware of his or her surroundings. This plant is on my top 10 list. It's an excellent tonic herb, strengthening the body in a gentle and consistent manner. It can be used safely by both adults and children and is readily available. For hay fever, it seems to have the most beneficial effect when used fresh. This is difficult, of course, because the nettle plant has tiny hairs on its aerial parts that contain formic acid—the same substance in bee venom and the constituent responsible for the contact dermatitis and pain when brushed against the skin. There are companies that freeze-dry the plant, assuring that most of the botanical substances responsible for the antihistamine effects are left intact and simultaneously removing the ability of the plant to "sting." This particular preparation is probably the best way to take nettle for hay fever symptoms. The recommended dose is 2 to 3 capsules three times a day.

Vitamin C also appears to have antihistamine properties, although research has been somewhat inconclusive. Most alternative health care practitioners recommend 1,000 to 3,000 milligrams of the supplement daily. Reactions to vitamin C are highly individual. I'm able to take fairly high amounts (5,000 milligrams a day) without problems, but I do this only occasionally. Generally, the current literature recommends taking vitamin C to "bowel tolerance," which means that if you begin to experience loose bowels or diarrhea concurrent with an increase in vitamin C consumption, you have taken too much. For the most part, people experience little difficulty with the dosage range noted above.

Another supplement that seems to beneficially affect hay fever is the bioflavanoid quercetin, especially if taken in conjunction with vitamin C. The recommended dosage is 400 milligrams of quercetin two to three times a day. Quercetin is not an inexpensive supplement, so if you don't notice positive results in a week or two, discontinue its use.

There are a number of homeopathic remedies on the market

that treat hay fever. As with most alternative remedies, their benefits vary from individual to individual. They seem to work quite well for children and are fairly safe, even for infants. However, I do recommend that if you wish to give your young child homeopathic medicine, it's best done under the supervision of someone trained in this modality.

As with many over-the-counter homeopathic remedies, it's possible to buy a formula that treats multiple hay fever symptoms, sort of the shotgun approach; or you can purchase individual remedies if you have specific symptoms you wish to treat and you know them precisely. If you're medicating yourself, the trick is to be able to match your particular set of symptoms to a specific remedy. While you can't really harm yourself if you choose the wrong remedy, results will be minimal and frustration high. If you have access to a homeopath, and your hay fever is severe, it might be wise to consult him or her first.

Hives

Hives are a reaction to an allergen that causes the body to create reddish welts, which itch terribly. Often the allergen is a food, but it can easily be any substance, including antibiotics and over-the-counter medications. In some cases the hives can spread over the entire body; left unchecked, they may spread to the respiratory system, making it difficult to breathe. In such a situation, which may be life threatening, medical treatment is required immediately. Do not try to treat a reaction of such severity yourself.

As with any severe itching, it's helpful to calm the body, psyche, and soul. A sedating nervine tea or tincture is useful at such a time. Try a calming tincture made from the following herbs: 1 part linden flowers (*Tilia* spp.), 1 part skullcap (*Scutellaria* spp.), 2 parts catnip *(Nepeta cataria),* 1 part lavender *(Lavandula angustifolia),* and ½ part peppermint *(Mentha* x *piperita).* See the section on making tinctures in chapter 1 for more information on how to make this yourself. Take 30 to 60 drops in a little warm water to begin with, and follow with 10 to 15 drops every hour until the itching stops. Five to 7 drops of lavender essential oil added to a warm bath will help calm the body as well.

A soothing paste can be made of green clay and water. Spread this mixture over the hives and allow it to dry. If you've made up some Drying Clay Poultice (see page 54) ahead of time and happen to have it with you, use this instead. The echinacea and goldenseal contained in it won't hurt, and you get another double-duty product. Some people find calendula creams useful as well. There are a number of such products commonly available on the market, and they can easily be carried in a travel first-aid kit.

Oats are particularly soothing to the skin. While rolled or cut oats supposedly no longer have calming constituents, I think I'd try slathering a cooled, runny oatmeal over hives if nothing else was available. When you're traveling, sometimes you have to think creatively and use what's at hand.

ANXIETY

Anxiety is the term used to describe feelings of excessive concern, worry, or panic. The range of emotions felt varies from situation to situation and person to person. Often the feelings appear to have no source—there seems to be no reason to be nervous, yet the fear persists. Anxiety can be accompanied by physical sensations, particularly as the level of anxiety increases. Examples are rapid heartbeat, sweaty palms, nervous stomach, muscle tension, dry mouth, and diarrhea. We've all felt this way before—when introducing ourselves at a company function, or prior to meeting our prospective in-laws for the first time (or fifth!). I must admit to an ever-increasing level of anxiety each time I fly. I grew up on airplanes, it seems, and I never experienced any fear. Now, as an adult, flying has become nerve racking at best. It's not the delays and inconveniences, although they probably contribute to the situation. It's a nameless fear of what might happen and an increasing belief that these jumbo, streamlined buses with wings shouldn't be defying gravity—they have no business doing so. I know this is irrational and so I fly, but not without my lavender essential oil, personal meditative routines, and mandatory glass of white wine.

There are also individuals who experience a very real and extreme sense of anxiety during what are commonly called anxiety attacks. There are good alternative therapies for this syndrome, including the remedies discussed below, but the subject is too broad for me to cover here.

There are a number of alternative therapies useful for anxiety, and all travel well. Herbally speaking, kava *(Piper methysticum)* is probably my favorite. Pharmacists believe that the pharmacological effects are due primarily to kavalactones, constituents found in the fat-soluble part of the root. This would explain why kava is traditionally served combined with coconut milk, a substance high in fat. The coconut milk makes it much more palatable as well!

Kava is a Polynesian island plant and was historically imbibed only by tribal royalty. Served in a traditional kava ceremony, it was often given to rival tribes who had come to talk treaty. Kava has a calming effect and promotes sociability. Since it engenders a pleasant sense of tranquillity, an alert mind, and no desire to hack apart tribal enemies, it became a very useful tool at such diplomatic occasions.

In addition to containing anti-anxiety properties, kava works as a sedative, analgesic, and muscle relaxant. Current studies indicate that it does not appear to work in the same way as benzodiazepines (a class of pharmaceuticals including Valium), in that kavalactones do not bind to the benzodiazepine receptor sites. You shouldn't mix kava with prescription anti-anxiety or antidepressant medication, however, unless you're under the care of a health care practitioner. Nor should kava be taken concurrently with alcohol.

Kava is most conveniently taken either in capsule form or as a tincture. I'll warn you—it has quite an interesting taste. As a member of the pepper family, it carries quite a "bite"— not so much a feeling of heat as one of numbness. If you don't relish the idea of having a numb throat, capsules will work best for you. The dosage depends on the percentage of kavalactones present in the herbal preparation. Used to fight anxiety, 70 to 85 milligrams of kavalactones would be appropriate. This would approximately correlate to a 250-milligram capsule containing 30 percent kavalactones. Harold H. Bloomfield, M.D., recommends starting with the dosage above in the evening. If this doesn't work, you can take another dose in the morning and add a third at midday if your anxiety continues. If you're like me and anxiety plagues you situationally, perhaps prior to flight, take a dose several hours before boarding, and another just prior to takeoff. Remember not to drink alcohol while taking kava. In addition, do not use kava if you have Parkinson's disease or are pregnant or nursing. One other warning: Some people have an adverse reaction to kava in the form of headaches that, in a few cases, can be quite severe. I suggest trying kava prior to traveling to ascertain your own reaction. Most folks have no problem at all.

Another excellent herb for anxiety, especially when it's chronic, is chamomile *(Matricaria recutita)*. Christopher Hobbs writes in *Stress and Natural Healing,* "Don't underestimate chamomile. It is considered a mild herb, but if you make a strong tincture or tea and take enough of it, it can produce miracles." Hobbs recommends 1 to 2 cups of chamomile tea, three times a day. He does warn, however, that a very strong tea can cause vomiting. I've never known anyone to have such a reaction to chamomile, which is often used to settle the stomach, so I believe it would have to be a very strong infusion indeed to produce such an effect. It's easy enough to pack chamomile tea bags in your carry-on luggage, or even to slip a few in your pocket. Most places will serve you a tea setup if you ask. As noted in the section on allergies, some individuals may be sensitive to chamomile, resulting in allergic symptoms. For more information, read the section on page 57.

Many of the same nervine herbs that are used to treat stress can be used as remedies for anxiety. They include valerian *(Valeriana officinalis)*, California poppy *(Eschscholzia californica)*, lemon balm *(Melissa officinalis)*, passionflower *(Passiflora incarnata)*, and lavender *(Lavandula angustifolia)*. Please read the sections on insomnia and stress for more information on these particular herbs.

As an alternative therapy, aromatherapy works extremely well when anxiety becomes an issue. Not surprisingly, a few of the same plants that are beneficial for anxiety when taken as herbal preparations are similarly useful in essential oil form. Both lavender and chamomile, specifically German chamomile *(Matricaria recutita),* are good examples. Do as your granny did and carry a cotton handkerchief dosed with 5 to 7 drops of lavender or chamomile. You can discreetly hold your hankie to your nose and take a few deep breaths. Having been intimately involved in the technological revolution of the late twentieth century, I admit that I demand predictable, noticeable results—now—with the emphasis on *noticeable*. I must say that essential oils don't necessarily comply. They are much more elusive and work their magic best when you aren't watching. So don't expect immediate relaxation after taking a sniff of your lavender handkerchief. Half an hour later, however, when you've forgotten the word *anxiety,* you may notice how much fun you're having—what a surprise!

You can also make a spritzer with your favorite anti-anxiety blend of essential oils. To do so, fill a 2-ounce bottle that has a spray top with distilled water and add 20 to 30 drops of essential oils, either a blend or a single oil. Simply shake and spray. My favorite mixture of essential oils to spritz when I'm stressed is 18 drops of lavender, 8 drops of sandalwood, and 4 drops of rose. Unfortunately, this is a costly blend. Real rose essential oil sells for more than $200 an ounce. Sandalwood is protected, and while it's not currently as expensive as rose essential oil, it's produced from the heartwood and roots of the tree, making it in many ways more dear. Please use it wisely and judiciously. Other essential oils that have proven useful for anxiety are bergamot (the essential oil used to flavor and scent Earl Grey tea), patchouli, marjoram, jasmine, clary sage, neroli, and melissa. For more information on their specific properties and uses, read Kathi Keville and Mindy Green's excellent and informative book, *Aromatherapy: A Complete Guide to the Healing Art.*

While an essential-oil-laced handerkerchief and spritzers are handy on the go, a warm footbath in your hotel room can also work wonders. Fill the tub partially with hot water—you're only going to sit on the edge and soak your feet. You can get away with a little more essential oil (10 to 15 drops) than what you'd normally use for a full bath, since feet (and hands) are a little less sensitive. Try 6 drops of lavender, 3 drops of peppermint, and 3 drops of bergamot. Read the room-service menu and dream about what you might eat in bed—with no one to tell you differently.

Rescue Remedy, a blend of five different flower essences discovered by Dr. Bach, is a natural for treating anxiety. If you're feeling anxious, try a couple of drops of Rescue Remedy either directly under your tongue or in a glass of water. If the anxiety persists, repeat the dose 15 minutes later, and continue every two to three hours throughout the day. You cannot overdose yourself with flower essences, but if one doesn't seem to relieve the symptoms within a day, it's not the "correct" essence for you. Pear flower essence, produced by the Master Flower Essence Company, may be used in similar situations as Rescue Remedy. If you're also using the spritzer mentioned above for treating anxiety, try adding 4 drops of Rescue Remedy to the blend for an increased effect. I once made a spritzer for work with lavender essential oil and Rescue Remedy. One day I organized a meeting between several of my internal customers and a vendor who was known to be particularly tough to deal with. Thinking ahead, I sprayed the empty room with the spritzer five minutes prior to the meeting. Within fifteen minutes, all participants had settled down and were cooperatively discussing the topic at hand.

Several other flower essences are traditionally used to alleviate anxiety. Aspen, in particular, is good for "anxiety that has no known reason." Mimulus is indicated for "excessive anxiety and nervousness about daily life," while the Mustard flower essence is recommended for anxiety in general.

Phosphorus, or Phos., as it is commonly labeled on homeopathic remedies, is a specific for anxiety. Symptoms that indicate its use are nervousness under pressure, a tendency to keep emotions inside, and a fear of illness or death. Dr. C. Norman Shealy, the author of *The Illustrated Encyclopedia of Natural Remedies,* notes, "As a homeopathic treatment, it is mainly given to those suffering from anxiety and digestive disorders." Take as discussed in chapter 3.

I have one last recommendation. Its beauty is that it can't be carried, only borrowed. I am speaking of your breath and its use as a tool for relieving anxiety. The next time you feel anxious, spend a few minutes "watching" your breath and posture. My guess is that your shoulders are lifted and hunched, and your breath is quick and shallow. You can fool your body by consciously creating the physical symptoms that are the hallmarks of a calm state. Begin by dropping your shoulders. Now, close your eyes and begin to take deliberate, slow breaths. Breathe in through your nose to a count of 4 and exhale to a count of 7. Take another breath in this manner, and then another. Continue slow, conscious breathing while focusing on the physical sensations this deep breathing brings. Within minutes, your body and mind will begin to relax. Try this when your plane is taxiing down the runway prior to takeoff.

ATHLETE'S FOOT

The bane of the athletic gym attendee, athlete's foot is caused by a fungus known as *Tinea pedis*. It causes burning, itching, and inflammation in and around the toes and on the feet. It spreads easily and is often picked up in public showers and damp floors, such as those in a gym bathroom. One way to prevent the infection is to wear bath shoes or waterproof sandals in a public shower or bathroom. The fungus likes to grow in damp, dark places—such as sweaty feet encased in socks and shoes. Therefore, one way to prevent or relieve a case of athlete's foot is to go around barefoot as much as is safe and possible. In addition, the use of drying remedies, such as vinegar- or clay-based products, is an excellent way to eradicate the infection.

A number of herbs and essential oils have antifungal properties. Garlic, berberine-containing plants such as goldenseal (*Hydrastis canadensis*) and Oregon grape (*Mahonia aquifolium*), usnea (*Usnea* spp.), and black walnut (*Juglans nigra*) hulls are all terrific for killing the fungus that causes athlete's foot. Tea tree, lavender, and clove bud essential oils can also be used. Both lavender and tea tree essential oils may be used neat—that is, dabbed straight on the toes and feet. Clove bud essential oil should be diluted in a bit of carrier oil before applying.

Athlete's Foot Treatment

The following protocol may be used to treat a case of athlete's foot while traveling or at home.

1. **Foot soaks.** Soak your feet in a basin to which you've added several cloves of crushed garlic, a bit of rubbing alcohol, and

some warm water. This should be done once daily for at least 5 minutes. Both garlic and rubbing alcohol should be readily obtainable in most countries if you do a bit of searching. An alternative is to use 10 to 15 drops of tea tree essential oil and 1 cup of salt. If you don't want to bother or don't have access to a tub or basin, skip this step.

2. **Foot powder.** After your foot soak or anytime you've had a bath, dust your feet with Athlete's Foot Dusting Powder (below). The powder contains herbs and essential oils with antifungal properties and helps keep the feet dry. You can put on socks at this point if you need to wear shoes.

ATHLETE'S FOOT DUSTING POWDER

You can make this up ahead of time and carry it with you in a clean spice jar that has a shaker top and lid. Sprinkle it on your feet and in your socks before putting on your shoes.

1. Place $\frac{1}{2}$ cup bentonite clay in a bowl—a small, deep bowl works best, because it's easier to stir the resulting mixture without the clay "dusting" your work area.

2. Add $\frac{1}{4}$ cup powdered black walnut hull powder and $\frac{1}{4}$ cup powdered Oregon grape root. I suggest buying both of these herbs already powdered, because it's difficult to powder them finely enough with the average coffee grinder. You definitely don't want a gritty foot powder on sore toes! Mix the powders with the clay.

3. Add $\frac{1}{2}$ teaspoon clove bud essential oil and $\frac{1}{2}$ teaspoon tea tree oil. Mix well to break up any resulting clumps.

4. Let the bowl sit, covered with a clean cloth, for a day. Then store the mixture in an airtight container.

BLEEDING

This ailment needs no description. The first-aid rules for stopping the free flow of blood are well known, but I'll summarize them here:

1. Bleeding results from a cut in either a capillary, a vein, or an artery. In the case of the first two, the bleeding will be slow. Arterial cuts are the most serious, because the blood flow will be rapid and startling. Death can result in a matter of minutes if the flow of blood is not arrested.

2. To stop the bleeding in all cases, a constant, firm pressure to the wound is required. A superficial cut that affects only the capillaries may require nothing more than a bandage.

3. For more serious, stubborn bleeding, place a clean gauze pad on the wound and apply even pressure. Kathi Keville suggests placing a credit card inside the gauze pad to facilitate more even application of pressure. If the wound is to an extremity, raise the limb above the heart. It's harder for the heart to pump blood to an area that is above it, and this alone will help reduce the amount of blood lost.

From an herbal standpoint, there are a number of herbs with hemostatic properties (they assist in stopping hemorrhaging and internal bleeding) and styptic properties (they reduce and stop external bleeding). These herbs work because of their astringent action and coagulating effects. Examples of such herbs are yarrow

(*Achillea* spp.), shepherd's purse (*Capsella bursa pastoris*), cayenne (*Capsicum* spp.), white oak (*Quercus alba*) bark, and goldenseal (*Hydrastis canadensis*).

Often, excessive bleeding can be fairly traumatic for both the person injured and those nearby. Remember that Rescue Remedy or Pear flower essence (see chapter 4) is an excellent remedy for emotional trauma and should be used for everyone involved.

Internal Bleeding

Internal bleeding, or hemorrhage, can be an extremely serious condition, and it's highly recommended that you seek professional help immediately to ascertain the extent of the injury. Nothing should be taken internally if the bowel has been perforated unless a qualified physician recommends otherwise.

On a less serious note, when I entered my forties I noticed that my periods began to come more frequently, and on occasion more heavily (due to small uterine fibroids). On one such occasion I found that I needed to change my tampon every fifteen minutes. I took 1 dropperful of Hemorrhage Tincture every fifteen minutes until the flow lessened, and I was able to continue with regular activity. The Hemorrhage Tincture may also be used for nosebleeds.

◆

HEMORRHAGE TINCTURE

1 part yarrow
1 part shepherd's purse

Use a standard method for making herbal tinctures described in the section on tinctures.

External Bleeding

In all cases, follow the first-aid protocol above. For superficial cuts that do not respond quickly to pressure, a powdered styptic herb may be the answer; it's wise to have several of these on hand. I keep powdered yarrow, cayenne, and goldenseal in my first-aid kit, because they're useful for a number of complaints. Sprinkle the herbal powder directly on the wound. Any of them will work to help coagulate the blood and astringe the area.

BLISTERS

Ouch—these do hurt! Try to be proactive and cover sensitive areas of the feet before putting on those hiking boots or shoes, especially if they're new or if you expect to be walking long distances. I've started carrying adhesive bandages around with me in my purse or pocket when I know I'm going to be on my feet for a while. The minute I feel any irritation at all, off come the shoes and socks, and on goes the bandage. My husband, a thirty-year Sierra Mountain backpacking veteran, once gave me some excellent advice: "Don't tough it out; there's no shame in stopping and taking a look at what hurts."

Moleskin, a soft fuzzy cloth with an adhesive backing, is an imperative if you're backpacking or trekking around in hiking boots. You can purchase moleskin in varying degrees of thickness, so shop around to see what might suit you best. If you have the room for it in your bags, it sometimes works well to have several different sorts. Follow the instructions on the package for application. You'll need scissors to cut it to the required size, so don't forget to take along a small pair. Many

Swiss Army knives include a tiny pair of scissors, which will work just fine.

What to do if you do get a blister? To begin with, resist the temptation to pop it. Doing so increases the risk of infection, and the blood serum (the fluid inside the skin pocket) helps keep the tissues clean and allows the injury to heal. Try to keep the blister dry and clean. A little aloe vera gel or calendula *(Calendula officinalis)* salve can be applied to the blister; top it off with a bandage. At night be sure to remove the bandage to allow the blister to dry.

If the blister ruptures on its own, or if it's severe enough for the skin to have been partially or completely rubbed away, put a few drops of Roman chamomile or lavender essential oil in a cup of water, stir, and apply to the open skin with a bit of cotton. An herbal antiseptic salve may be applied afterward, before you bandage the wound. The priority here is to keep the blister clean, which may mean changing bandages and reapplying salves throughout the day.

That same husband who gave me such good advice forgot to take it himself and ended up with two severe blisters on each heel. So he could complete a lengthy backpacking trip that had been in the planning for months, we devised a complicated procedure for his blister management. Both morning and evening he removed the bandages, cleansed the blisters with soap and water and hydrogen peroxide, and applied an antiseptic salve. To bandage the blisters, he cut pieces of gauze the size of each blister and placed them over each wound. Over these he placed a relatively thick moleskin that had been cut in the shape of an elongated doughnut, the center hole exactly matching the piece of gauze. Next came another piece of moleskin, thinner this time, which lay whole over the first layer. This setup created a clean, protected area over each blister. It also took quite a long time to complete and wouldn't be my first recommendation, but he was out in the middle of nowhere and something had to be done. If you do get blisters, the best possible remedy is to stay off your feet as much as possible and let them heal (so to speak!).

BLOODY NOSE

Nosebleeds have a number of sources and can be fairly dramatic. Generally a broken capillary is the culprit, from either a cold or hay fever. As with other types of bleeding, pressure applied to the bridge of the nose works best. The common approach used to be to tilt the head backward to keep the blood from coming out of the nose. However, this just causes the blood to drain to the back of the throat and, in a severe nosebleed, may cause choking. Current thought recommends lowering the head to the knees and maintaining pressure on the bridge of the nose. A cold compress can also be used. Soak it in cold water to which several drops of lavender essential oil have been added to help with trauma.

BRUISES

A bruise, technically known as a contusion, is caused by a blow to the body resulting in broken capillaries, which leak blood to surrounding tissues. Left to heal on its own, a bruise will generally disappear in a few weeks. Sometimes unexplained bruising is due to a deficiency in vitamin C.

One of the best herbs for healing a bruise is arnica *(Arnica montana)*. This tall, mountain plant bears daisylike yellow flowers.

Available as a tincture, it is recommended for external use only, except in very small quantities and then only under the supervision of a knowledgeable herbalist. The exception to this is when arnica is taken as a homeopathic remedy. Because it is present in such minute amounts in a homeopathic dose, it causes no toxicity.

Apply arnica cream, salve, gel, or homeopathic spray to any area of the body that has been banged up for any reason. You can also make an arnica compress by adding 60 drops of arnica tincture to 1 cup of warm water. Soak clean gauze or a cotton cloth in the solution and then apply it to the injured area. Leave in place for 20 to 60 minutes. Do not apply arnica to broken skin, which will cause undue irritation, unless it's in the form of a homeopathic spray.

Internal doses of homeopathic arnica may be used in addition to topical remedies. You can buy homeopathic arnica at your health food store. An appropriate strength is 30x (or 30c). Internal homeopathic remedies are taken either as tiny pellets left to dissolve under the tongue (sublingually) or as liquid drops.

Bruising can also be relieved with St. John's wort *(Hypericum perforatum)*. Apply St. John's wort oil directly to the skin. One advantage this herb has over arnica is that it can be applied safely to broken skin, as long as the area has been cleansed first.

If you prefer, try an essential oil compress. Using the same method as for arnica, above, soak a clean piece of gauze or a washcloth in 1 cup of warm water to which 5 drops of essential oil have been added. Use lavender, chamomile, or geranium essential oils, either singly or as a blend. Apply the wet cloth to the bruise for as long as you or the patient will allow, ideally 20 to 60 minutes.

BUG BITES AND STINGS

Summer would not be complete without reminders from the insect world that we humans are not alone in the outdoors. A simple remedy for bug bites and stings is to gently tie a slice of onion in place over the site; this can work wonders. There are a number of other natural steps to take as well.

The rule of thumb with a bee sting is to ensure that the stinger has been removed—otherwise the bee's irritant will continue to enter the skin. Look for the stinger immediately after being stung and scrape or pull it out. Some people have severe allergic reactions to bee stings. If you begin to have problems breathing, develop hives, or the site of the sting becomes quite swollen and infected looking, be sure to see a health care practitioner at once.

Plantain (*Plantago* spp.), which grows all over the North American continent and is often unwelcome in suburban yards, makes an excellent topical remedy. It comes in both broad-leaved (*P. major*) and narrow-leaved (*P. lanceolata*) varieties, and the two work similarly. Plantain is composed of tannins, which are astringent in action and will help relieve any sting as well as reduce any itching and swelling. To use, choose several leaves and either macerate (chew) them to make a "spit poultice" or chop them finely to produce a pulpy mixture. This can then be applied as a poultice to the bite or sting. Cover with gauze and tie in place. Relief should arrive within 15 minutes. Fresh chickweed (*Stellaria media*) also works well as a quick-relief poultice. Make sure that you're comfortable identifying both these plants before using them, and don't chew or use any that have been sprayed with insecticide or herbicide.

Another remarkable remedy is Drying Clay Poultice (see the recipe on page 54). Just dab it onto the bite or sting and let it dry. The lavender essential oil relieves itching and stinging, the echinacea-goldenseal tincture prevents infection, and the clay draws out toxins. This paste can also be used on infected insect bites.

Speaking of lavender essential oil, it's also very effective used alone on insect bites and stings. Beause it's one of the few essential oils that can be applied directly to the skin without being diluted, just place a few drops on your finger and rub it onto the bite or sting. Lavender essential oil relieves pain and inflammation and has antibacterial properties as well. Peppermint essential oil, which has an immediate cooling effect, is also a wonderful remedy for bee stings Because peppermint oil has a rubifacient action (stimulating blood flow), the chemicals in both the bee venom and those produced by the body as a reaction to the sting will quickly be carried away.

If the bite or sting becomes infected, take echinacea (*Echinacea* spp.) tincture. Usually ¼ teaspoon in 1 cup of warm water several times a day will do the trick. For more stubborn infections, goldenseal *(Hydrastis canadensis)* or osha *(Ligusticum canbyi)* tincture is effective. I like to use small doses of 5 to 10 drops more frequently—every one to two hours. If an infection doesn't clear up in a week, or if it worsens, seek professional care.

Sometimes insect stings take a long time to resolve. In this case try taking echinacea-goldenseal capsules every three hours. The reaction should discontinue within a couple of days.

BUNIONS

A bunion is really a form of bursitis, an inflammation of the bursa, and in this case settles in at the soft tissue surrounding the base of the big toe. It appears that women are more prone to the affliction than are men. One of the causes is badly fitted shoes. Given the fact that women, more than men, wear abominable shoes for the sake of fashion, it doesn't surprise me that we end up with more bunions.

In addition to ensuring that shoes fit properly, it helps to go barefoot as much as possible. If you're traveling a long distance by air or in a bus or car, remove your shoes and replace them with some heavy-duty comfortable socks. The idea is to relieve any prolonged pressure to the base of the toe.

Because chamomile *(Matricaria recutita)* is a strong anti-inflammatory, drinking its tea several times throughout the day will help relieve some of the pain. If you're using chamomile tea bags, you might try placing one directly on the bunion as a kind of poultice before tossing it in the garbage. St. John's wort *(Hypericum perforatum),* an herb that works directly on neural tissue, can be taken both internally as a tincture and externally in the form of an oil or salve rubbed directly on the bunion. If you're using the tincture, try 30 drops three times a day. This herb can increase photosensitivity in humans, although you seldom hear of any problems. Taking it for a short duration—three weeks or less—shouldn't pose a threat. Take it longer than that and it might be wise to limit your exposure to the sun.

Chamomile and lavender essential oils—both useful for many external pains—can effectively relieve the inflammation and discomfort associated with bunions. While lavender can be applied directly to the foot, chamomile essential oil should be diluted in a bit of vegetable oil prior to application. Mix 5 drops of chamomile essential oil with 1 ounce of carrier oil. Gently massage a bit of the resulting oil into the bunion several times a day and before retiring.

BURNS

My all-time favorite burn remedy is lavender essential oil applied neat. It can work magic on minor burns. One Christmas, I decided to make peanut brittle candy. As I was pouring the boiling syrup on the cookie sheets, a bit dropped on my antique oak table. Without thinking, I scooped it up with my finger. The pain was sudden and intense. A deep blister immediately began to form, and I rushed to put my finger under cold running water. After letting the cold water run on my finger awhile, I dried it, coated it well with lavender essential oil, and put on an adhesive bandage. Within only fifteen minutes, the pain was mostly gone and by the next morning the burn seemed to have resolved itself. It never did blister and I lost no skin.

Still, herbal remedies are best left for first-degree burns; more serious burns should be treated professionally, especially if they're large. However, there are a number of good herbal treatments for less severe burns. To begin with, always cool the burn by letting cold water run over it or by immersing it in a cold-water bath for a minute or more. Then you can apply a topical remedy to relieve pain and speed the healing process. Although many of us were brought up to apply butter to a burn, current thought indicates avoiding oil-based products unless the burn is very small.

Many people practice herbal first aid each time they use aloe on a small kitchen-related burn. My mom keeps a small aloe plant in her kitchen that she uses frequently . . . unfortunately! To use the aloe plant, simply snip off a bit of a leaf, open it up lengthwise, and apply the cool gel inside to the burn. You can also buy aloe gel or products especially for burns containing aloe in the health food store. Make sure the product contains a high percentage of aloe—at least 90 prercent.

I make a salve that works well on burns. I like to use it after the heat has subsided—maybe a day later. To make it, follow the general instructions for making salves in the section on oils and salves.

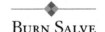

Burn Salve

¹/₃ cup fresh plantain
¹/₃ cup calendula
¹/₆ cup chamomile
¹/₃ cup lavender buds
¹/₆ cup rosebuds
¹/₃ cup comfrey leaf
2 ¹/₂ cups olive oil
2 ounces beeswax
1 tablespoon lavender essential oil

Make an herbal oil with the herbs. After straining, add the beeswax to the warm oil (you may have to reheat the oil a little so that the beeswax can melt—or, if you're using melted beeswax, so that it doesn't curdle). Once you have tested for the correct consistency, add the lavender essential oil, stir well, and pour the mixture into little jars.

If you don't want to make your own salve, there are many on the market that are similar to the one above. Look for plantain (*Plantago* spp.), calendula *(Calendula officinalis),* St. John's wort *(Hypericum perforatum),* aloe, and comfrey *(Symphytum officinale)* as ingredients. You don't need them all—just a few.

St. John's wort oil is an effective treatment for burns once the heat has subsided, especially combined with an herbal oil of dandelion blossoms. The common dandelion blossom *(Taraxacum officinale)* is an excellent anodyne, bringing pain relief. Next time, pick your dandelion blossoms for medicine rather than cursing and spraying them!

Believe it or not, another great remedy for burns is cold black tea. My great-aunt Mollie, a nurse in the Philippines in the early 1920s, learned about ice tea and burns while on duty there. I got to try it out when I singed my calf on the exhaust pipe of a motorcycle. We happened to be at a burger joint, so I got a large glass of iced tea and poured it slowly over the burn, which was about the size of a silver dollar. I don't necessarily recommend this, but the nurse in the emergency room did say that the burn looked clean and was healing very nicely. It appears that the tannic acid in black tea restores the acid balance of the skin while helping the proteins in the top layers of the skin form a kind of protective covering.

Sunburn

Despite all the warnings we get to stay out of the sun, people still manage to overdose. For the most part, use the same types of treatment noted above for burns. Aloe gel stored in the refrigerator is soothing applied to parched, sunburned skin. Or make a pleasant spritzer with 1 cup distilled water, $\frac{1}{2}$ cup aloe gel, and $1/2$ teaspoon lavender essential oil. Just put the mixture into a spray bottle and use.

Herbal baths are also wonderful for sunburn because you can totally immerse the body and soak for a while, giving the herbs more time to work. For herbal baths, I usually make a really strong infusion on the stove and then add it to the bath. Good herbs for sunburn would be comfrey *(Symphytum officinale),* lavender *(Lavandula angustifolia),* plantain *(Plantago* spp.), and calendula *(Calendula officinalis).* A time-honored remedy for sunburn is an apple cider vinegar bath: Just add a cup of apple cider vinegar to the bathwater and soak. Apple cider vinegar acts in much the same way as black tea, restoring the natural acid balance to the skin.

As sunburn begins to heal, it can often leave behind dry, flaking, and itchy skin. The emollient and soothing properties of oats come to the rescue here. Try an oatmeal colloidal bath such as Aveeno to help soothe and stop the itching. Oats have a gentle nervine action and will calm the whole person, inside and out.

CONGESTION

People get congested for all sorts of reasons, most commonly due to colds and flu or allergic reactions. While the treatment for congestion is largely the same regardless of the cause, it's important to know the reason so that treatment can be extended appropriately. One major difference between herbal medicine and standard, allopathic medicine is *what* gets treated. Most of us have been raised in a medical system that goes directly for relieving the symptom, leaving the source untreated. This can create a vicious cycle wherein the root cause is driven deeper into the body, producing recurrent bouts of symptoms and weakening the overall system.

One of the reasons the body produces excess mucus is to help rid itself of whatever is causing the problem. Most herbalists and holistic practitioners assert that drying up mucus interferes with the body's natural healing response. I agree with this, but I also feel that there are occasions when too much congestion and mucus serves only to further weaken the body. In these cases—pneumonia is an extreme example, as is traveling by air, when you must withstand extreme changes in air pressure—it may be appropriate to use pharmaceutical decongestants.

Steam Inhalations

Steam inhalations are one of the most effective natural ways to relieve respiratory congestion. The warm steam helps ease difficult breathing, while volatile oils from herbs and essential oils have both decongestant and antibacterial actions. Inhalations act in accordance with the concept of supporting the body's healing powers by helping clear mucus rather than dry it up.

To make an herbal steam inhalation, fill a 2-quart saucepan half full of water. Add $^{1}/_{2}$ to 1 cup of your chosen herbs, cover, bring to a boil, turn off the heat, and let sit for 10 to15 minutes. After the herbs have steeped, the steam inhalation is ready. You may also add up to 6 drops of essential oils at this time, if desired; if you don't have any dried herbs, you can use the essential oils only. They are equally effective. Place the pan on a towel or place mat on a table. Sit with your head over the pan, then cover your head and the pan with a towel to create a tent. It's best to keep your eyes closed so they don't burn. Breathe the herbal steam slowly, taking care not to get too close to the hot water. You can regulate the amount of steam and temperature by opening and closing the towel. Steam for 5 to 10 minutes.

It's recommended that steam inhalations be repeated three to four times a day when you're congested. One note of caution: Don't use steam inhalations when you're suffering from an asthma attack, or if you have rosacea, broken facial capillaries, or sunburn. Also, steam inhalations will cause the mucous membranes to be sensitive for a period of time, so it's best to not go out right away.

Good herbs to use are eucalyptus *(Eucalyptus globulus)*, peppermint *(Mentha* x piperita), thyme *(Thymus vulgaris)*, pine needles, rosemary *(Rosmarinus officinalis)*, and chamomile *(Matricaria recutita)*. You can use these in any combination. The essential oils of any of the aforementioned herbs would be helpful, as well as tea tree, hyssop, and lavender.

Portable Inhalations

Since it may be difficult to muster up a steam inhalation in remote areas or when you're staying in a hotel, a portable inhalation can be used instead. You can buy these at your health food store. Olbas makes a great one that's light and takes up little room. Or you can make your own quite easily from a small jar with a tight-fitting lid, some rock salt, and essential oils. Simply fill the jar with rock salt and add enough essential oil(s)—30 to 40 drops—to get a good whiff of the scent when you hold the open jar to your nose. Keep the jar tightly capped when not in use to prevent evaporation of the essential oils. Use the same essential oils recommended in the section on steam inhalation, above. You might also add some dried rosemary *(Rosemarinus officinalis)* to the rock salt mixture before putting it in the jar.

A good herbal vapor salve rubbed into the chest before sleeping can also help. You can buy such salves or make your own. If you do make your own, you'll find that it's important to use more essential oil than you normally would when scenting herbal salves, in part because the essential oils evaporate as they're added to the warm oil mixture. A guideline is 2 tablespoons of essential oils to 1 cup of olive oil. For the essential oil blend, try 2 teaspoons of peppermint essential oil, 1 teaspoon of rosemary, 2 teaspoons of eucalyptus, and 1 teaspoon of thyme (chemotype linalol). To make, heat the olive oil and add ¾ ounce of beeswax. When the beeswax has melted, stir in the oils and pour the salve into small jars to harden. Cap immediately to prevent further evaporation of the essential oils. You can also use 1 cup of herb-infused olive oil in place of the plain olive oil; see the section on oils and salves for directions. Rosemary and thyme are good herbs to use in the infusion: Both are high in beneficial volatile oils and have antibacterial properties.

COLDS AND FLU

Everyone has their own favorite cold remedy. Mine is my husband's chicken soup. The good news is that most countries have their own version of chicken soup—all you have to do is inquire. Better yet, if you feel well enough to dine out, ask what the host recommends. You might come back with a new remedy!

The truth is that cold and influenza viruses are constantly present around us. We're exposed to them daily and remain healthy because our immune systems are working as they should. There are times, however, when our systems don't respond effectively due to stress, not getting enough sleep, lack of exercise, poor eating habits—all hallmarks of travel. Sometimes a cold is nature's call to slow down and take care of yourself. Whatever you can do to nurture yourself or your family will help when someone has a cold.

Start by boosting your immune system. Echinacea became the panacea of the 1990s, and for good reason. It stimulates the immune system and helps the body rid itself of microbial infection. It's worth remembering that because of echinacea's popularity, the plant has been overharvested to the point of endangerment. On the positive side, echinacea is easy to cultivate, and it's now possible to buy organically cultivated echinacea. *Echinacea angustifolia* and *E. purpurea* are equally effective, and many products contain *E. pallida* as well. Start taking echinacea tincture—30 to 45 drops three times a day—a week before traveling to obtain its immune-enhancing effects. While all treatments work differently, depending on the individual, experience shows that echinacea can knock out a cold if taken at the *onset* of symptoms. To do so, I prefer frequent doses of echinacea tincture throughout the day—generally 30 to 45 drops every hour. If the cold symptoms don't abate within two days, you can assume that the cold is here to stay for its duration. But don't stop taking the echinacea. At this point, you can reduce the dose to 30 to 45 drops three times a day; there's a good chance that your cold will be gone more quickly than if you had given up on treatment.

Another effective immune-enhancing formula is a combination of astragalus *(Astragalus membranaceus)* and Siberian ginseng *(Eleutherococcus senticosus)* taken as a tincture twice a day, 20 to 30 drops per dose. This formula is appropriate to take daily throughout the cold and flu season. Begin a month prior to travel.

An herbal remedy that I've recently become quite fond of for both colds and flu—because it works *really* well for both my family and me—is a tincture of equal parts boneset *(Eupatorium perfoliatum),* redroot *(Ceanothus* spp.), and echinacea. Boneset, like echinacea, is an immune stimulant. Stephen Harrod Buhner explains in his informative book *Herbal Antibiotics* that boneset "increases phagocytosis to four times that of echinacea." Phagocytosis is the process by which a certain form of phagocyte—macrophages, to be exact—go about the body devouring assaulting bacteria. After an infection, the macrophages perform internal housekeeping by cleaning up white blood cell remains as well as leftover bits of bacteria. I've seen them likened to Pac Man. You may not have heard much about boneset because it hasn't become trendy . . . yet. But in the 1700s and 1800s most U.S. homes in the Northeast had boneset drying from the rafters. It was used effectively to treat a flu epidemic in Pennsylvania in 1800. Matthew Wood hypothesizes that the name *boneset* referred to the pain that "set" in the bones when a person had the flu.

Redroot is an equally effective botanical, especially for stimulating and cleansing the lymph system. The lymph system is responsible for processing and cleansing the body of the by-products of fighting infection. That's why health care practitioners always check the lymph glands in your neck when you're ill: Swollen lymph glands are a sign that your body is working to rid itself of infection. The faster the lymph can rid itself of cellular debris, the faster you'll recover from a cold or flu.

While I don't believe that this boneset-redroot-echinacea

formula is available for purchase yet, you can easily make it yourself. Buy single-herb tinctures of each of the three herbs and combine them in a larger jar. Fill a 2-ounce tincture bottle with some of the resulting formula and you're all set. Be sure to label both jar and bottle. As with echinacea, I like taking this remedy fairly frequently—generally 20 to 30 drops every hour—at the onset of a cold or flu. Once symptoms begin to subside, reduce the dose to 30 to 45 drops, three times a day until you're well.

A standard remedy for flu is the homeopathic formula Oscillococcinum. Manufactured by Boiron, Oscillo (as it's often called) is available even in the more progressive grocery stores these days. It's taken like any other homeopathic remedy— sublingually (allowed to dissolve under the tongue) 30 minutes before or after eating or drinking anything except water. The standard dosage is three vials; each vial contains hundreds of minute pellets. As soon as you feel flu symptoms, take a vial of Oscillo. Repeat with the second vial six hours later, and with the third six hours after the second. Oscillo is a great remedy for travel because of its tiny size. The vials will easily fit in a purse, pocket, or first-aid kit.

I can't help but mention what has become the "old standby"— vitamin C. Though still controversial, studies and experience show that large doses of vitamin C begun as soon as you feel a cold coming on will reduce the severity and length of related symptoms. The recommended dose is 1,000 milligrams every two hours for the first several days. Some people tolerate vitamin C less well than others; for them, such a high dose may cause diarrhea. If this occurs, reduce the dosage until the diarrhea has subsided. Alternative remedies for other cold- and flu-related symptoms such as coughs, sore throat, and fever are discussed in their own sections.

CONSTIPATION

For me, constipation is the expected result of any travel. Often the result of not drinking enough fluid and not getting enough exercise—that sounds pretty much like air travel to me—constipation can all but ruin a trip. You can help prevent it by drinking a lot of water (make sure it's either bottled or safe) and walking daily. Even then, the bowels have a tendency to slow down, especially if you're camping out and sleeping on the cold, hard ground. They don't like that combination one bit!

To get things moving again, try cayenne (*Capsicum* spp.). It's gentle and works effectively. Stir $\frac{1}{2}$ teaspoon of powdered cayenne into half a glass of water and drink the whole thing before bedtime. If things don't pass in the morning, take another dose. Cayenne is one of those items that does double duty (see the section on bleeding) and it takes up little room, so it's a natural for your first-aid kit. Similarly, eating a few local hot peppers will also work.

Cascara sagrada *(Rhamnus purshiana)* is another botanical laxative that many find effective. Its most easily taken as a capsule; follow the dosage instructions on the bottle. I find that cayenne works more consistently for me, but we each have different constitutions, so use what works. I advise starting with the lowest recommended dose of cascara and working upward until you obtain results. Also, find ways to include more fiber in your diet. It sounds obvious, but it may be harder to do if you are on a tour with set meals. If you trust the source, fruit will help. If not, take psyllium, a natural bulk laxative. There are a number of psyllium products available at either your drug or health food store.

A delightful remedy for constipation is a tummy massage. It

feels nicer if you can get someone to do it for you, but it's just as effective if you perform it yourself. Massaging with a few drops of chamomile essential oil diluted in vegetable oil further enhances the effect. The idea is to rub gently in circular, clockwise motions around the navel and outward, following the natural movement of debris in the large intestine. Try this for five minutes before going to bed. This also is very relieving for bouts of gas.

COUGHS

What I find most distasteful about getting sick is coughing. Annoying and debilitating, it is one of the ways our body rids itself of infection. Unfortunately, there really doesn't seem to be anything out there that will stop a cough dead in its tracks, even of the pharmaceutical variety. Well, codeine works pretty well to stop spasms, but that's about it.

An herbal cough syrup is your best bet. There are a number of them on the market; one flavored with elderberry (*Sambucus nigra*) can be helpful for its stimulating effect on the immune system. Otherwise your choice depends on the kind of cough you are treating—dry and hacking or wet and rattling. Many times you'll experience both during a bout with a cold, so it's good to either have two different kinds of cough syrup—one for each type of cough—or a syrup whose herbs work on both.

For a dry and hacking cough, often the more debilitating, demulcent and antitussive herbs are needed. Examples of herbs with demulcent (soothing) properties are marsh mallow root (*Althaea officinalis*), licorice root (*Glycyrrhiza glabra*), and mullein (*Verbascum thapsus*). The extraordinary-looking mullein plant is a specific for all lung complaints and can be used quite safely.

Licorice is one of my favorite herbs for its many differing actions and uses for a number of complaints, but it's contraindicated for those suffering from edema or high blood pressure. Botanicals that reduce coughing (antitussive) include lobelia *(Lobelia inflata)* and wild cherry *(Prunus serotina)* bark. Valerian *(Valeriana officinalis),* while not specific for coughing, has antispasmodic and sedative properties; it takes the place of codeine (without the side effects and risk) in a natural cough remedy. If you're making your own cough syrup and decide to include lobelia, be judicious with the amount you use. Lobelia is a "power" herb and can cause vomiting, even in small amounts. Additionally, the plant is on the United Plant Savers At-Risk List and is becoming increasingly difficult to find in the wild.

When your cough becomes "productive"—wet and rattling—expectorant herbs may be used to clear the mucus. Elecampane *(Inula helenium)* is a favorite of mine, not only because it works so well but also because of its statuesque beauty. Mullein is useful here, as are hyssop *(Hyssopus officinalis)* and eucalyptus *(Eucalyptus globulus).*

Herbal steams made with either plant material or essential oils will deliver the helpful plant constituents directly to the lungs. See the section on congestion for more information on how to prepare an herbal steam and on contraindications. I find steams especially useful when my cough is wet and productive. Herbal steams should be used with caution if you suffer from asthma. Many essential oils are irritating in such cases.

I find herbal cough drops or lozenges to be helpful when trying to suppress a cough; these can be purchased all over the world. The sucking and delivery of herbal saliva down the back of the throat can be very soothing.

CRAMPS

Nothing is worse than a charley horse (intense muscle cramp) in your leg when you're sitting in a restrictive seat on the plane. The pain is sudden and intense and usually happens without warning. Possible causes include mineral or hormonal imbalances, sore muscles, or too much blood getting into the muscle. Relief can be had by vigorously massaging the muscle along its length and with the fibers. Massage the area for several minutes, until the blood is moving well and the cramping has ceased.

Stretching also works well. I often feel a cramp coming on in my feet when I'm sitting in certain yoga positions. The only cure is to unfold and stretch my toes in the opposite direction from what they were in. Heat, in the form of a hot-water bottle or heating pad, is not recommended; it serves only to bring more blood to the area. Try elevating the limb instead.

Certain supplements can be helpful, depending on the reason for the cramping. I find that if I'm in a hot climate and perspiring a lot, muscle cramping becomes a common occurrence. Eating salty foods helps. Don't increase your salt intake, however, if you have high blood pressure or edema, don't tolerate it well, or have been told by your health care practitioner to avoid sodium. Recently, certain football teams have begun drinking pickle juice—high in salt content—as a preventive measure for cramps.

Vitamin E is sometimes suggested for charley horses that occur at night due to circulatory problems. The recommended dosage is 600 International Units (IUs) of vitamin E daily for two weeks; then reduce this to 400 IUs daily. Menopausal women with frequent nocturnal cramping should start their daily vitamin E dosage at 1,200 IUs. After two weeks, the dosage should be reduced to 400 IUs. Magnesium and calcium deficiencies may also contribute to cramping. Try eating more of the foods rich in these minerals, including cold-water fish (halibut, mackerel), spinach, kale, pumpkin seeds, and tofu.

CRANKINESS

When I get cranky, my husband says that he needs to either "water" me or "air" me out. Kind of like being a mattress! But he's really referring to the benefits of hydrotherapy and fresh air. And as much as I don't want to admit it, he's right—it always works!

So if crankiness is a problem, especially in little ones, the first thing to do is let them take a nice warm bath with a few drops of lavender or chamomile essential oil thrown in. Adults can do the same or take a shower, if one is available. If you're showering, place a few drops of one of the essential oils mentioned above on a hot terry washcloth and hold it near your face (eyes closed) as the steamy water drums against your skin. Upon exiting the tub or shower, briskly dry off with a fluffy towel—it's a new day.

If a bath or shower is not available and you have the time, go for a quick, brisk walk. Deep breathing helps clear out stuck chi (life force) and a bit of exercise will get your blood pumping, both excellent for dispelling "bad attitudes." It will also give you a taste of the local flavor, which can give you a new sense of life.

Another favorite remedy of mine—which I don't indulge in too often because of its expense—is rose essential oil. Refer to chapter 2, Aromatherapy, and you'll understand why. The number of rose petals needed to produce just an ounce of the essential oil is huge. Still, rose essential oil not only smells heavenly but also has the ability to restore calm and peace. And a little does go a long way. Try putting just 1 drop on a cotton hankie and breathing deeply of the scented material. You'll soon find your sense of joy returning. Rose essential oil is safe for children as well.

One last remedy, and perhaps the most effective, is Dr. Bach's Rescue Remedy. Discussed in chapter 4, Flower Essences, Rescue Remedy works to dispel crankiness as well as trauma. Try 4 drops under the tongue several times a day. If your infant is the cranky one and you've taken steps to understand the cause and have addressed it, it also helps to place a few drops of the essence on your hands and rub them gently over your baby's scalp and temples. Babies often respond remarkably quickly.

CUTS, SCRAPES, AND ABRASIONS

Unfortunately, traveling and being away from home doesn't mean you might not take a tumble and get a scraped knee, or worse. However you come by an injury of this sort, it's especially important to cleanse the wound well when you're in a different environment than you're accustomed to. Different locations mean different bacteria and a need to be extra vigilant. It's good to know that in people with normal clotting abilities, some bleeding is beneficial: It's the body's way of ridding itself of harmful foreign matter. If you've got a superficial cut on your finger, for instance, you might want to squeeze out a bit of blood under the water faucet to help your body cleanse itself. The main point is to wash the wound completely. Soap and warm water work very well. If you have no access to water, slowly pouring a little hydrogen peroxide on the cut or abrasion also helps cleanse the area. Follow up with a good herbal antibacterial liniment. I like Dr. Kloss's Liniment, which can be easily made at home. The recipe can be found in Dr. Kloss's classic *Back to Eden*. It contains goldenseal, cayenne, and myrrh, and employs old-fashioned rubbing alcohol as the menstruum. On an open wound this solution burns and stings and is not for the faint of heart. I definitely recommend diluting it with some sterile water before using it on children or animals. Be careful not to get any of the liniment on your clothing—the goldenseal imparts a yellow-gold color to the solution, and it will stain. If you prefer not to make your own Kloss's Liniment, most health food stores carry some type of herbal liniment for cuts and scrapes.

Once the wound has been washed and disinfected, apply a salve that contains both soothing and antibacterial herbs. Particular herbs to look for are chickweed *(Stellaria media)*, plantain *(Plantago* spp.), goldenseal *(Hydrastis canadensis)*, St. John's wort *(Hypericum perforatum)*, lavender *(Lavandula angustifolia)*, thyme *(Thymus vulgaris)*, osha *(Ligusticum canbyi)*, usnea *(Usnea* spp.), and calendula *(Calendula officinalis)*. Remember not to use arnica *(Arnica montana)* on broken skin, and stay away from external remedies containing comfrey *(Symphytum officinale)* until the wound has developed a good scab and shows no signs of infection. While comfrey is an excellent demulcent and especially healing to the skin, its ability to help the skin repair itself quickly can seal infection-causing pathogens deep in the wound. A good commercial salve for traveling is the Golden Salve, made by Paul Strauss, herbalist, caretaker of Earth, and owner of Equinox Botanicals in Rutland, Ohio. After applying the salve, bandage the wound as appropriate.

One last remedy to consider is Herb Pharm's Propolis/ Echinacea Spray. It can be used for numerous complaints, which earns it a spot in my first-aid kit. As the product name suggests, one of its ingredients is propolis, a by-product of the honey industry. A resinous material that bees produce to help seal off their hives from bacteria and other infection-causing material, propolis is a truly natural antibiotic. Spraying it on a scrape or abrasion creates a protective covering, just like the bees get for their hives. The other ingredients in the spray are antibacterial and immune enhancing and will further help the wound heal.

CYSTITIS OR URINARY TRACT INFECTION

A urinary tract infection, often abbreviated as UTI and some-times referred to as cystitis, is an inflammation of the urinary tract caused by an overgrowth of bacteria and resulting in infection. Sometimes referred to as "honeymoon disease," it's more common in women than in men. This is due to anatomy— a man's urethra is approximately 8 inches in length, while most women have a urethra measuring 1 1/2 inches. This means that bacteria have less distance to travel to reach the bladder. Symp-toms of a UTI are frequent urination, pain, spasming and burning while urinating, and sometimes fever and nausea if the infection is severe enough. It can be treated successfully with alternative methods, but if you don't get definite results within twenty-four to forty-eight hours, it's important to see a medical practitioner as quickly as possible. Left untreated, a UTI can lead to kidney infection. This is a serious condition indeed, and not to be taken lightly. Having said that, let me describe some of the alternative remedies you can try.

The first is prevention. UTIs are often the result of unsanitary conditions; of use of spermicides, diaphragms, feminine hygiene products, or antibiotics; and of stress. All serve to upset the internal balance. In women, it helps to wipe from front to back after moving the bowels, so as not to distribute bacteria from the rectum to the vaginal area, where the urethra is siutated. Another trick is to urinate prior to engaging in intercourse and especially afterward. The stream of urine passing through the urethra will remove much of any bacteria pushed up the urethra during intercourse. I've known women who all but eliminated recurrent UTIs by instituting both practices.

If you find yourself experiencing cystitislike symptoms while away from home, start drinking as much water as possible. Use bottled water if you are at all unsure of your water source. Drinking a lot of water will provide a steady flow of urine, which will allow more bacteria to pass from the system. Unsweetened cranberry juice is a time-honored treatment. Research shows that a constituent found in cranberries makes it difficult for bacteria to stick to the lining of the urethra and bladder. If the taste is too tart for you, dilute it with water. Drink at least three or four 8-ounce glasses a day. If you're prone to cystitis, you might want to take along cranberry capsules. These may be purchased at your health food store. The suggested dosage is 3 capsules containing 400 milligrams of cranberry extract every day until the infection is gone.

Herb Pharm produces a tincture called Goldenrod Horsetail Compound that I've found quite effective for UTIs. As the name suggests, it contains goldenrod *(Solidago canadensis)*, corn silk *(Zea mays)*, horsetail *(Equisetum arvense)*, pipsissewa *(Chimaphila umbellata)*, and juniper berry *(Juniperus communis)*. All of those herbs are specific to the health of the urinary tract. Some are more soothing and tonic in nature, such as corn silk, while others—juniper, for instance—have antimicrobial properties. The suggested dosage for an acute infection is 30 to 40 drops in water three to five times a day.

On a personal note, I once found myself displaying early UTI symptoms. Beer was readily available and as I knew I needed to drink a lot of fluids, I decided that the beer would have to do. I only drank two bottles, and the amazing thing was that my cystitis symptoms completely cleared themselves. I am not necessarily recommending beer as a natural treatment for cystitis—my guess is that the increased urination produced by drinking beer probably eliminated any offending bacteria—but if no other remedies were easily had, I might try it again.

DEHYDRATION

Dehydration is a condition in which the water level in the body falls below normal and the balance of electrolytes (sugars and salts) is upset. Causes include diarrhea, heat, air travel, exercise, and any situation where water isn't replaced in the body. Under normal circumstances, you're made aware of impending dehydration by a strong urge to drink fluids. But some people, especially many adults over the age of sixty, have a diminished awareness of dehydration due to age and certain medications (diuretics taken for heart disease and high blood pressure). These people need to manage their fluid intake by drinking at least six to eight glasses of water a day, depending on the environmental conditions.

Initial symptoms of dehydration include dry mouth, dizziness, loss of appetite, fatigue and weakness, and headache. These symptoms can occur even before thirst becomes a factor, so it's especially important to watch for them in children and the elderly when traveling in hot climates. Advanced symptoms include rapid pulse, vision and hearing problems, difficulty walking, and shortness of breath. Extreme dehydration is a serious condition and can result in death, so it's important to react quickly when you notice the signs.

As with many conditions, prevention is your best medicine. While plain drinking water is best for resolving dehydration, most other fluids will do as well, including juice, milk, herbal teas, and soft drinks. Six to eight 8-ounce glasses of water or a substitute are required each day—more if you're in a very hot area. Soft drinks are high in sodium, which will help retain water in the body, but they don't really quench your thirst. Stay away from them if they contain caffeine, which often acts as a diuretic. If you're in an area where the drinking water is suspect, bottled water, caffeine-free sodas, and canned or bottled juices may be your only recourse. Drinks with diuretic properties such as alcohol, coffee, and black tea are not appropriate in this situation, because they will further exacerbate the condition. Eating plenty of fruits and vegetables will also help; most contain at least 75 percent water.

Stay cool if possible. It's also important that when you're indoors there's plenty of air circulation. A hot, stuffy room is disaster for someone already suffering from dehydration. If air-conditioning is not available, numerous cool showers will help. If you're backpacking or camping, cool, rushing streams are an ideal place to soak your feet—or whole body, if you can manage it.

The main point is to try to replace the water in your body throughout the day. Drink frequently—at least every other hour, and more often if you're on an airplane. If you or someone in your party does become dehydrated, get out of the heat and drink fluids immediately.

DIARRHEA AND VOMITING

While it's not always the case, diarrhea and vomiting often go hand in hand, particularly when you're traveling. Intestinal disorders are all too common in unfamiliar areas, depending on what your body is used to and what it finds "foreign."

For most of us, used to years of effective sewage treatment in the United States, travel abroad poses some problems, especially if we drink the local water or eat unpeeled fruit or uncooked vegetables. And it can be difficult to eat without doing at least one of the three. To prepare yourself, Lois Johnson, M.D., suggests strengthening your digestive system by taking acidophilus and bifidus for several weeks ahead of time and while you travel. Often referred to as probiotics, acidophilus capsules (often with bifidus) can be purchased at your health food store. Take them in the morning, half an hour before eating. There are two types—one that must be refrigerated, one that needn't be. Either type works, and while I find the first more effective, you'll want the nonrefrigerated type for travel.

Dr. Johnson also suggests Para-Gard as a preventive measure. Para-Gard contains berberine sulfate, Citricidal extract, gentian root, goldenseal, Sweet Annie, quassia, black walnut hull, and garlic. It's considered a broad-spectrum herbal antimicrobial and is made by Tyler. Take 1 to 3 capsules three times a day between meals. Contact your health care practitioner for more information.

The Chinese patent remedy Curing Pill, discussed in the section on indigestion, is helpful for diarrhea and vomiting. If you suspect food poisoning, activated charcoal tablets would also be appropriate—see the section on food poisoning.

One of the most important concerns with diarrhea or vomiting is the possibility of dehydration. Try to replace the fluids that are lost by drinking small amounts of bottled water. This may be more easily said than done. If you're vomiting, sip small amounts of flat Coca-Cola or 7-Up. Sucking on ice chips, if they can be found, seems to work as well. Once you feel well enough, you might want to try some instant miso soup to help replace the electrolytes lost when ill. Be sure to see a professional health care practitioner if you have any of the following: severe dehydration, bloody diarrhea, or a fever higher that 100 degrees F.

EARACHES

Earaches are often a sign of ear infection, which can be a serious condition. Left untreated, it can result in perforation to the eardrum and hearing loss. At best, earaches and infections are incredibly painful.

Ear infections can be the result of blockage to the eustachian tube, which normally allows fluid from the middle ear to drain into the recesses of the throat. Blocked, this fluid becomes a breeding ground for bacteria and turns into pus and an infection. If it's preceded by a cold, an ear infection is referred to as a secondary infection. Causes of eustachian tube blockages are swollen glands or swollen tissue due to a cold, irregularities in the eustachian tubes (children born with cleft palates often have crooked eustachian tubes as a result), and allowing babies to drink from a bottle while reclining (bottle propping).

Holistic prevention includes eliminating dairy products, which lead to greater amounts of mucus in the body. It's also important to treat congestion—from colds or allergies—either with herbal steams or by taking a decongestant. I'm a fan of taking Sudafed before flights if I'm experiencing congestion. Flying increases pressure in the ear, and if you're already congested, it seems to drive the fluids deeper. I've ended up with an ear infection on more than one occasion from flying while sick. Chewing on gum or sucking on hard candy or a throat lozenge will also help relieve the pressure by opening up the eustachian tubes.

Dr. Kathi J. Kemper, in her book *The Holistic Pediatrician,* indicates that in most cases it's all right to treat an ear infection with alternative methods for up to twenty-four hours before contacting a health care professional. However, if the child is less than a year old, has a temperature of 103 degrees F or greater, is in severe pain, or seems to be sicker than would be normal, consultation with a health care professional is required as soon as possible. I would do the same for an individual of any age.

I have to admit that I have yet to find any of the typically suggested alternative treatments to be effective for earaches. Some people swear by garlic–mullein flower oil, although the one time I used it I ended up with a double ear infection that was incredibly painful. If this is something you'd like to use, treat both ears, even if only one seems to be problematic. To use the oil, warm it gently in a bowl of hot water, then put 2 drops into each ear. Be sure to keep the dropper itself from touching any area of the ear. Place a bit of cotton in each ear to keep the oil in place. Gaia Herbs offers this oil in a 2-ounce bottle that would pack well.

Two other alternative treatments for an earache that results from swimming or an infection in the ear canal (outer ear) are isopropyl alcohol and eardrops made from glycerin, grapefruit extract, and tea tree oil. Such drops can be purchased at a health food store. A company called NutriBiotic manufactures the ones I carry. Be sure to follow the directions on the bottle. Isopropyl alcohol works by drying up fluid stuck in the outer ear canal, which may be causing pain by putting pressure on the eardrum. To use, just place a few drops of alcohol in the ear canal, then put a cotton ball gently in the ear.

EYE PROBLEMS

This section focuses on dry eyes, puffy eyes, and conjunctivitis, commonly called pinkeye. Watering, itchy eyes due to allergies or hay fever are discussed in more detail in that section.

Dry eyes are often the result of irritants in the air, such as cigarette smoke, or a dry environment such as the desert or an airplane. Rehydrating your eyes will help. First, remember to drink lots of water, especially in an airplane: High altitudes will suck the water right out of your body. Cool compresses placed over both eyes will soothe and give them a rest. Don't use essential oils in the compresses—just soak clean gauze pads in ice water. Gently squeeze the water out and place the pads on your eyes. Leave them in place for 10 to 15 minutes. Natural eyedrops may be purchased at the health food store. These are often just saline solutions, but you might find some that also contain eyebright *(Euphrasia officinalis)*—an herb specific to eye complaints in general. Eyedrops are appropriate for traveling and symptomatic relief, but if you find that dry eyes are a common occurrence for you, consult your health care practitioner to determine if there isn't something else going on.

Puffy eyes can be a result of allergies, crying (maybe someone is a bit homesick), or too much partying. Relief is only as far away as your tea bag. When you're done drinking your tea, give your puffy eyes a break and place the tea bags directly over your closed eyes as a makeshift compress. Black tea contains tannins, which have an astringent quality, and will gently tighten the skin around your eyes by drawing out excess fluids. Another kitchen remedy—cold, sliced cucumbers placed over your eyes—works similarly. In addition, cucumber has emollient properties and will soften and soothe the delicate tissues around the eyes.

Conjunctivitis, or pinkeye, is an infection of the eye, such as a cold, which causes the cornea to become bloodshot. There may be irritation and a weepy discharge. The infection is often caused by a virus, but it can also be brought on by pollution or allergies. Despite its rather alarming appearance, if left untreated pinkeye usually resolves on its own. Still, there are some things you can do to relieve the discomfort and keep from passing on the virus:

1. Give yourself a break from eye makeup if you wear it. Using mascara brushes can pass the infection from one eye to the other and, worse yet, cause you to reinfect yourself later.

2. Use cold compresses to relieve the irritation.

3. Keep the eye clean. If oozing is a problem, you'll want to wash away the discharge. Use a clean washcloth wrung out in warm

water. Gently remove any debris from the eye. Make sure no one else in your family or traveling party uses the washcloth.

4. Don't wear contacts. They'll feel irritating and will keep the infection in place.

5. Keep your fingers out of your eyes as much as possible. While it might feel good at first to rub them, it will only irritate the eyeball further, and can also pass the infection from one eye to the other.

FATIGUE

Broadly speaking, fatigue is inevitable at some point in your travels. To begin with, you're spending long hours sitting in a cramped car, train, or airplane to arrive at your destination. Once you're there, the whirlwind begins, especially if you've opted for a guided tour. Then you sleep in an unfamiliar bed or, more difficult, on the ground. Even (or especially) if you're having a wonderful time and seeing exciting, exotic locales, travel leads to fatigue that, left unchecked, can easily become full-blown exhaustion.

Lois Johnson, M.D., once noted that if you wake up tired, you need to sleep more. It's just common sense: If you're beginning to feel fatigued, take a break. This can be especially difficult if you're traveling on business and other people's expectations of you are high. Think "balance," even if the word is unheard of in today's fast-paced business culture. It is possible to say no politely, and if you're feeling tired, do so. You'll have a more productive trip because of it.

Fatigue is often a result of not being able to relax. Insomnia and jet lag don't help either (see those sections for specific information). Exercise is a great way to reduce stress and relax. Many hotels all over the world have exercise rooms and pools, either right in the facility or through an affiliation with a local club that guests can use. It pays to make use of these if you need to de-stress. One of my coworkers is a veteran traveler and always goes for a jog when he arrives at his destination—even after thirteen hours in an airplane and two in a train. He claims that it both helps him sleep and allows him to eat whatever he wants! If running isn't your style, try a brisk walk instead.

On the sybaritic side, don't forget a warm bath with your favorite essential oils added just before you climb in. Good ones to relieve fatigue are rosemary, peppermint, clary sage, and lavender. Use them singly or in combination, but keep the total amount of essential oils down to 10 drops or fewer per bath. Peppermint essential oil is especially uplifting in the morning. Place a drop or two on a wet washcloth and breathe deeply from it while you shower.

Remember to eat well—whole foods and lots of water. Caffeine and sugar, while stimulating at first, will drop you hard later in the day. They can also mask fatigue by constantly jump-starting your system. Too much alcohol will disrupt your cycle and rob you of sleep (so desperately needed), so try to keep your drinking to a minimum—admittedly hard to do in Napa Valley!

FEVER

Fever, an internal body temperature above 98.6 degrees F, is a sign that the body is fighting off an infection. In fact, many health care practitioners don't consider a raised temperature a "fever" until it rises above 99.5. If it's not too high, a fever can be a good thing, because it's the body's way of destroying infectious pathogens. Many health care practitioners specifically advise against lowering a raised temperature, preferring to let it to run its course and do its job, unless it's prolonged or rises beyond 101. In these cases a fever can be debilitating. If it reaches 102.6 degrees or more, a fever can be quite serious indeed; if it's very high or doesn't go down within twelve hours, seek medical attention. Also consider the age of the individual—a temperature of 103 is not uncommon in young children but would be very difficult for an elderly person to tolerate.

Catnip *(Nepeta cataria)*—yes, the same plant that cats go bonkers over (it's a stimulant for them)—works well to alleviate fever. It's especially effective for children and can be used quite safely. Many holistic practitioners recommend a catnip enema for young children with fever (a room-temperature catnip infusion is used in the enema), but this may not be practical when you're traveling. Drinking the tea will have a similar effect; it can be made more palatable by adding peppermint *(Mentha x piperita)* leaf. The tea is equally useful for adults as well. To make the tea, infuse 1 to 2 teaspoons of catnip or catnip-peppermint herb in 1 cup of hot water. Let it steep for 15 minutes before drinking.

You may also want to make or buy a tincture containing herbs that act as a febrifuge (able to reduce a fever) to carry in your kit. I make one containing 2 parts catnip, 1 part elder flowers *(Sambucus nigra),* and 1 part peppermint. This particular tincture is especially useful if the fever is due to cold or flu.

Peppermint and lavender essential oils are very soothing in a cold compress. Add 2 to 4 drops of essential oil to a basin of cold water. Soak a washcloth in the water and wring it out. This can be placed either on the forehead or at the nape of the neck (I like to rotate between both areas); it's quite relieving. Change the compress every 10 minutes or as often as needed.

Cool baths may be required if someone's temperature is quite high and you're unable to get to a health care practitioner right away. Adding 5 to 7 drops of lavender essential oil to the bath will help calm the patient. And stay close—it's entirely possible that he or she will require assistance out of the bath. Also, be on the lookout for chills and make sure to dry the person well once out of the tub. I also recommend a dose (4 drops under the tongue) of Dr. Bach's Rescue Remedy every hour or two—more often for someone who's quite uncomfortable.

If the fever is severe or prolonged, dehydration can become a factor. While people generally don't feel like drinking while feverish, insist that little sips be taken often. Ice chips are also a pleasant way to get fluids into the body under such conditions. If your attempts at reducing a fever—with either these methods or over-the-counter analgesics such as Tylenol or aspirin—are not successful, or if it's quite high given the guidelines noted earlier, seek professional care immediately.

FOOD POISONING

Food poisoning can occur anywhere, but it does seem that your chances of it increase in more remote locales. Symptoms include dizziness, vomiting, diarrhea, nausea, intestinal cramping, sweating, and possibly a low fever. You know when you have it, and if you've had it before you also know that it needs to run its course. There are, however, a few things you can do to help relieve the symptoms.

One of the easiest is to eat bread, if you can get past putting solid food in your stomach. The bread will help soak up the toxins and allow you to pass more of them faster. Don't use spreads on the bread, however. They'll just make you feel more ill.

Activated charcoal, which can be purchased in tablet or capsule form, has been found to be very effective in cases of food poisoning. The charcoal is extremely absorbent, not only of toxic particles in the digestive tract but also of gases. As the charcoal passes through the digestive system, it picks up offending toxins and other wastes and is excreted along with the "poison." Activated charcoal is sold most often in doses ranging from 250 to 350 milligrams and can be purchased at your health food store. Read the label for proper dosage.

There are also a few homeopathic remedies that you can try. Since they're relatively inexpensive, you might want to buy both and have them on hand, just in case. If you're experiencing nausea, vomiting, diarrhea, chills, and restlessness, try *Arsenicum album* in either 6C or 12C potency. Take a dose every two to three hours until the symptoms subside. *Veratrum album,* 6C or 12C, may be used if the symptoms are similar but accompanied by a craving for ice-cold drinks and cold sweats. Again, doses may be taken every two or three hours.

Food poisoning can be quite severe and may require medical attention. If the patient is a very young child or elderly, seek help immediately upon the onset of symptoms. This also holds true for those suffering from a chronic disease such as AIDS. If symptoms include a temperature over 100 degrees F; bloody diarrhea; an inability to keep down any fluids; dehydration; difficulty in breathing, speaking, or swallowing; paralysis; or change in vision—or if symptoms are more minor but last longer than twenty-four to forty-eight hours—seek medical attention immediately.

HEADACHE

A headache can ruin even the most delightful occasion, or at the least put a damper on it. Interestingly, in the alternative world (as compared with the over-the-counter world) treatments often depend on why the headache has occurred. And while you'll find a number of holistic remedies for headaches that are general in nature, it's important to note and assess what was going on prior to the onset of the headache so that the cause may also be addressed.

For instance, I often get headaches if I've become dehydrated. In fact, if I complain of headache, the first thing my husband asks is, "How much water did you drink today?" Simply drinking a glass or two of cool water and finding some mild activity with which to occupy myself usually clears the headache.

For other people, stress may be the cause of a headache or perhaps sinus congestion due to allergies. Both conditions have specific treatments, and using them not only helps relieve the headache but will also keep it from returning. Migraines are a different animal entirely and have specific treatments—feverfew *(Chrysanthemum parthenium)* appears to be successful for some—but the focus of this section is on your garden-variety headache.

One of the first alternative headache treatments I experienced was at the hands of a young Japanese woman at a New Year's Eve party. I mentioned that I had a headache—probably from drinking too little water and more than enough alcohol. She took my left hand in hers and began to vigorously massage a point on the web of skin between my thumb and forefinger. Called the *he-gu* point in acupuncture, stimulating it serves to release congested chi (vital energy—a concept critical in traditional Chinese medicine and other healing modalities) and relieve aheadache. It works, but remember to treat the source as well. In this case I also needed to drink more water. To find the point yourself, hold your hand palm down with your thumb resting against the side of your hand. With a finger from the opposite hand, locate the point where the crease made by the thumb resting against the hand ends. Keep your finger on this point and allow your thumb to move outward. You'll find that you've located a point on the skin between the forefinger and thumb. It's found on both hands, and both work equally well.

Another excellent remedy is lavender essential oil. Not only does lavender relax, but it also has analgesic properties. You can use it in a spritzer (see chapter 2, Aromatherapy, for instructions on how to make one) or, better yet, place a drop or two on your fingertips and massage them into the base of your skull at the back of your neck. I also like to massage it into my temples if the headache seems to rest there. Keep in mind that just as when you're using ibuprofen or aspirin, your headache won't dissipate immediately; with a bit of time, however, it will begin to subside and eventually disappear. If you have access to a tub, take a steamy lavender bath (add 5 to 7 drops to the bathwater), close your eyes, and relax.

HEAT EXHAUSTION AND SUNSTROKE

Heat exhaustion can occur when the body becomes overheated, generally from being out in the direct sun without protection, for a prolonged amount of time. If left untreated, sunstroke may occur, which is much more serious than heat exhaustion and requires immediate medical attention.

Symptoms of heat exhaustion include dizziness, weakness, and clammy skin. Sunstroke, on the other hand, will include a high fever, racing pulse, and no sweating at all. If this occurs, again, immediate medical treatment is required.

To mitigate heat exhaustion, it's important to rehydrate. Give water in frequent, small amounts. In addition, lost minerals and salts must be replenished. This can be accomplished by drinking fruit juices, sports drinks such as Gatorade that are designed to replace the body's electrolytes, broths, and miso soup. Kathi Keville notes that she began to keep instant miso soup packets in her first-aid kit after experiencing heat exhaustion herself. This is an excellent idea—and the packets are perfect for backpacking, when weight is an issue.

Cool showers or baths may be taken, if possible. If not, make cold compresses using washcloths dipped in cold water to which you've added a few drops of lavender essential oil. These can be placed at the forehead, temples, and other pulse points on the body. Growing up in Libya, I often ran cold water from the school's bathroom tap over my wrists when I was hot. Somehow I knew it would cool me down.

INDIGESTION

Travel includes all sorts of events that can upset the digestive balance, causing bloating, indigestion, or heartburn. Stress plays a huge part, as do the unusual foods we tend to eat while abroad. Luckily, a number of natural remedies are not only easy to carry but also usually quite effective in relieving and eliminating indigestion.

Bloating, a full, rather uncomfortable feeling in the abdominal area, is often a result of digestive disturbance and stress, which are themselves frequently a result of overeating or eating foods that your body is unused or sensitive to—especially if you're consuming more sugars and starches than is normal for you.

In many Indian restaurants a small bowl of fennel seeds is placed near the entrance. Those in the know will take a small spoonful of the seeds and eat them as they leave. Fennel *(Foeniculum vulgare)* has carminative properties and works to relieve flatulence as well as stimulating digestion. Carry your own small tin of fennel seeds with you to chew after meals—only a few are needed. They have a delightful taste and will leave your breath smelling fresher as well.

Another suggestion is chamomile *(Matricaria recutita)* or peppermint *(Mentha x piperita)* tea. Both herbs relieve gas and indigestion. Peppermint is classified as a stimulating nervine but will soothe the nerves in the digestive tract, which will help eliminate any accompanying cramping. Carry tea bags of both types and use as desired. I like the two plants combined in equal parts as a tea blend—it's simple and flavorful. Just take some along in a plastic bag with a tea ball, and all you'll need is hot water. Use 1 to 2 teaspoons per cup, depending on your tastes. Let the tea steep for 5 to 10 minutes before drinking.

Children in particular will respond favorably to a gentle tummy rub with vegetable oil and a few drops of essential oil. You can purchase 1-ounce plastic bottles and make up any number of essential oil blends to take with you. Make sure to label the bottles—most of us can't trust our noses. Pack each bottle in a plastic bag to avoid leaking oil over the rest of your belongings.

Tummy Oil

To relieve uncomfortable bloating, gently rub some
Tummy Oil on the abdominal area. The essental oils
smell good and will help to the whole area.

2 drops lavender essential oil
1 drop sweet fennel essential oil
2 drops German chamomile essential oil
1 ounce sweet almond, apricot kernel, or grapeseed oil
  (plain vegetable oil also works)

Bitters Blend

Bitters, discussed in the section on allergies, are wonderful
for relieving heartburn. Used half an hour prior to eating,
bitters will prevent indigestion by stimulating the body's
gastric secretions at the appropriate time—just before you
load your stomach with food. If you want to make your
own bitters tincture, try this recipe. There are also many
similar products on the market—just ask the staff at your
favorite health food store to help you pick one.

2 parts dandelion root
¹/₂ part gentian root
1 part cardamom
1 part fennel
1 part chamomile
1 part gingerroot
¹/₂ part turmeric

Grind the herbs and mascerate in 80-proof brandy for
two to six weeks. Refer to the section on tinctures for
additional information.

Finally, a Chinese patent remedy called Curing Pill is truly excellent for any kind of digestive disturbance, including nausea. My brother-in-law offered it to me once after we had eaten a rich meal and I was feeling badly. Curing Pills come prepackaged in a small plastic vial that contains approximately one hundred tiny reddish brown pills. The idea is to swallow them all down at once with water. I must admit to having been dubious and somewhat reticent to swallow a bunch of pills, no matter how little. But within a half hour, I felt well. Now I always carry several of the little red boxes, each containing one plastic vial or dose, in all my kits. You never know when you'll need one. You can buy ten individual boxes in one larger box at most health food stores—or try a local acupuncturist (I note that mine says "Culing Pill"—it's the same thing.)

INSOMNIA

The bane of the long-distance traveler who jumps time zones in a single bound, insomnia also torments many of us on a regular basis. The causes are varied and difficult to pinpoint—in fact, each healing modality sees the causes very differently—but it's known that stress often plays a part.

And insomnia can indeed be a factor when crossing many time zones. The body's clock is "set" to a particular time, so when it suddenly finds itself in a totally different time of day, it's thrown off. Sleep habits are then disturbed, which may cause temporary insomnia. Camping, too, can make it difficult to sleep. I have yet to find a pad that feels as good as my bed; I never sleep well outdoors.

A number of herbs work effectively for treating insomnia. My favorite is valerian *(Valeriana officinalis),* in spite of its infamous musty—read "smelly socks"—odor. Valerian contains constituents that have sedative and hypnotic properties. The term *hypnotic* in this case means "something that induces sleep." It can be taken as a tea: Leave 1 to 2 teaspoons of root per cup of hot water to steep for 15 minutes. Even though it's the root that gets used, the tea is prepared as an infusion so not to lose the beneficial volatile oils. If you find the peculiar valerian odor offensive, the herb is equally effective taken as a tincture or in capsule form. Lois Johnson, M.D., indicates that valerian may be taken safely even in fairly high doses; she's taken as much as a tablespoon of the tincture at night when sleep was elusive. I recommend starting off with smaller doses—1 to 2 droppers approximately half an hour before retiring—to see how the herb works for you. You can increase the dosage if need be, although I don't recommend going beyond a tablespoon of tincture. Valerian will make it easier to get to sleep and won't cause a "hangover" the next morning, as do some pharmaceutical sleep remedies. One thing to keep in mind is that in 5 to 10 percent of the population, valerian has the opposite effect, acting as a stimulant. There really are no indicators to let you know if you're a member of that minority; the only way to know is to try it. I've been told that if valerian *is* a stimulant for you, you'll have no doubt about it.

Although valerian is known as the primary "sleeping" herb, other herbs also have sedating, calming properties, are safe to use, and can be equally effective. Skullcap *(Scutellaria laterifolia)* is considered a nervine tonic and sedative. It's especially effective in those suffering from nervous tension. Catnip *(Nepeta cataria)* and lemon balm *(Melissa officinalis)* are both gentle, relaxing herbs and are often found in children's formulas. Passionflower

(Passiflora incarnata) is an incredibly beautiful plant with both sedating and hypnotic actions. David Hoffmann recommends it for "intransigent insomnia"—cases of insomnia that are well established. Hops *(Humulus lupulus),* the same plant used to flavor beer, is also considered a sedative and hypnotic. It has a bitter flavor and is contraindicated in those who are also suffering from depression. Most herbal formulas for insomnia contain some, or perhaps all, of the herbs listed here. In particular skullcap, valerian, and hops combine well. Your best bet is to talk with the folks at your health food store and let them recommend a favorite product—there are plenty available.

Keep in mind the foods you may be eating as well. Beverages or foods containing caffeine will make it more difficult to sleep. That innocuous piece of chocolate left on your pillow as part of many hotels' turndown ritual contains caffeine. Small as the piece may be, if you're at all sensitive to caffeine, it will be enough to keep you awake. Many over-the-counter formulations also contain caffeine—certain pain relievers are a good example—so be sure to read the labels.

Ever-useful lavender essential oil also has calming, sedating properties and has been successfully used to aid sleep. I find that just 2 or 3 drops on a tissue placed inside my pillowcase will help bring on a relaxing sleep. Taking a warm bath to which 5 to 7 drops of lavender oil have been added just before you go to bed is also effective. Don't let the water get too hot or you may find yourself somewhat agitated instead.

Melatonin is a natural hormone that many find useful when dealing with insomnia. The recommended dose for insomnia is 1 to 3 milligrams taken an hour or two before bed. It's discussed in more detail in the section on jet lag.

ITCHINESS

A common problem while traveling, itchy skin obviously has a number of sources, but several in particular come up when you're away from home.

Itchy skin can occur when the outer dermal layers become dry. Every winter I suffer from intermittent itching when my office and home are heated and the air's moisture content is all but removed. It's especially bad when I bend my arms or legs—the stretching of dry, taut skin increases the itching. I've discovered that in winter I need to moisturize my whole body, not just my face. Airplanes are also particularly drying due to the high altitudes and recycled air. To help keep your skin from drying out, keep your insides moist by drinking lots of liquids, especially water, while flying. If there's any one thing that can be done to counteract the rigors of flying, whether jet lag or dry skin, it's to drink enough water. A good rule of thumb is one glass (airplane sized) of water every hour.

Calendula *(Calendula officinalis)*—sometimes called marigold, although it's not the same as the garden marigold commonly found at nurseries—has anti-inflammatory properties and is specific to skin care. Products made with calendula are extra soothing on dry, chapped skin; I use oil infused with calendula in most of the soap I make. If you find that your skin is getting dry and itchy, try massaging a lotion or cream made with calendula into your skin. When shopping at the health food store, you might look for a lotion that also contains chickweed *(Stellaria media),* which has both vulnerary (relieves pain) and emollient properties.

Cool compresses made with a few drops of Roman

chamomile, peppermint, lavender, or eucalyptus essential oil added to the water will also help. Just take gauze pads or a washcloth, wring them out in cold water to which 2 or 3 drops of essential oil have been added, and place them over the itching skin. Don't use hot water: Heat will cause blood to rise to the surface, which will only increase the itching.

Sometimes severe itching is due to stress or inflammation and needs to be calmed internally. If you have valerian *(Valeriana officinalis)* tincture in your first-aid kit, take 30 to 60 drops in a small glass of warm water. Chamomile *(Matricaria recutita)* tea is also useful. Besides being very calming, it has a strong anti-inflammatory action. Some children become quite anxious when they're itchy. Rescue Remedy will effectively calm them down. Let them sip water or chamomile tea to which 4 drops of Rescue Remedy has been added. In fact, you can also buy Rescue Remedy cream. Massage them, or yourself, with this cream for both a moisturizing and a calming effect.

JET LAG

Jet lag is the name given to the collection of physical symptoms that arise when you fly across time zones. Flying west seems to be easier on the body, but whether your flight takes an easterly or westerly direction and depending on the distance flown, jet lag will likely result. While it's not a particularly serious condition, jet lag does interfere with normal activity. A hallmark symptom is the inability to sleep at night—your body's time clock as been thrown off, so when it's 11:00 P.M. in Amsterdam, you may feel like it's midafternoon, not bedtime. Additional symptoms include fuzzy headedness—an inability to think clearly—fatigue, weakness, irritability, and dehydration. Actually, the dehydration is generally due to flying at high altitudes without drinking enough water or other hydrating fluids. It contributes to the severity of jet lag. So one of the golden rules for avoiding or lessening jet lag is to drink plenty of fluids (not alcohol or sodas) while flying. See the section on dehydration for additional information.

Experts agree that resetting your internal body clock is imperative. Eating according to the time of your destination can help with this. For example, you arrive in Rome at 10:00 A.M. Your body thinks it's one o'clock in the morning—you would prefer to be sleeping. By the time you clear customs and arrive at your aunt and uncle's house, it's 12:30 P.M. and your aunt has prepared an incredible meal. *Mangia!* Eat! Not only will you make your aunt happy, but your body will begin to think that it's actually lunchtime. Yes, you're still tired, but because you fooled your body by feeding it according to the hour, your adjustment to the new time zone will occur more quickly.

Lavender and peppermint essential oils can also come to the rescue. Think of lavender as the evening essential oil and peppermint as its morning counterpart. This is a rough rule of thumb, of course, and not to be taken too literally. Still, both essential oils are considered to have nervine properties—they act directly on the nervous system. Because lavender essential oil has a relaxing, mildly sedating action, you may prefer to use it at night when your want to coax your body and mind to slow down and sleep. Peppermint stimulates and would be appropriate to use in the morning instead of a cup of coffee. If you don't have peppermint essential oil, rosemary can be substituted. Lavender can also be used in the tub, though peppermint might be a little too irritating for a bath. Place a few drops on a hankie instead, and breathe deeply. Using the oils in this manner, one at night and the other in the morning, again helps you reset your inner clock.

Melatonin is a natural hormone produced in the pineal gland of the brain; it helps regulate human circadian rhythms (the body's clock). Around midevening the pineal gland secretes melatonin for several hours, which lowers your internal temperature and readies you for sleep. Melatonin can be used to reset your internal clock when traveling by using the following protocol. Begin taking 5 milligrams of melatonin each night an hour or two before bed for three nights before your trip. Take it again (5 milligrams) the night of your arrival. You may find that you need to take it for several nights afterward, as well. The recommended dosage for insomnia is 1 to 3 milligrams, so I don't recommend taking the 5-milligram dose for very long.

One final tip: this comes from a dear friend with whom I had the pleasure of working for several years. Several of us had flown to London on a business trip and we arrived at our destination at 10:00 A.M. My friend explained that the only "sure cure" for jet lag consisted of two very specific things. First, we had to stay awake all day—no naps that would inevitably turn into a full night's sleep. One was to walk about the town or go to the office. Easy choice, that one! The second item—the "active ingredient"—was one's dinner. My friend explained that we must "go out for curry." This didn't just mean that we ate curried vegetables somewhere. It meant that we spent two hours partaking of a full Indian meal and then washed it down with a bottle of Indian beer. I admit I was dubious at first, and then delighted with the meal, but best of all, I slept a full nine hours that night and awoke refreshed and ready to go the next morning. In the years since, I have tried to rationalize this phenomenon by believing that it was a just a case of setting our internal clocks. But truthfully, I think it was the magic of the curry and being with friends.

MENSTRUAL CRAMPS

Sometimes referred to as dysmenorrhea, which really means "painful menstruation," menstrual cramps have been experienced by most women at some point in their lives. Interestingly enough, it wasn't until fairly recently that the medical establishment recognized cramps as real; previously it preferred to classify the complaint as psychosomatic.

Nutritional modification can help alleviate cramping, but it should be continued for a period of time to be effective. Evening primrose oil—take two 500-milligram capsules three times a day—will help by affecting prostaglandin levels, which in turn affect inflammation and pain. Sometimes cramping is due to calcium or magnesium deficiencies. Eating more dark, leafy greens such as spinach, chard, and kale will help, as will eating almonds and sesame seeds. If you feel more comfortable taking supplements, the recommended dosages are 800 milligrams of calcium and 1,000 milligrams of magnesium taken nightly.

For situational relief, movement helps. Try walking, stretching, or yoga (inverted positions are not recommended while menstruating). Amanda McQuade Crawford recommends the following: Lying flat on your back, bring your knees to your chest and rock gently back and forth. This particular movement will apply gentle pressure to the lower back, where cramping is often felt. It also promotes blood flow in the pelvic region.

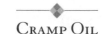

Cramp Oil

Essential oils are particularly useful for painful cramping. This blend can easily be made ahead of time and placed in your first-aid kit.

> *1 ounce sweet almond oil (infused with dandelion flowers is a plus, since they are pain relieving)*
> *4 drops lavender essential oil*
> *4 drops clary sage essential oil*
> *2 drops ginger essential oil*
> *2 drops marjoram essential oil*

Lavender relaxes, ginger warms, marjoram is an antispasmodic, and clary sage is a specific for menstrual pain. To use, shake the container to disperse the essential oils in the carrier oil, pour a small amount into your hands, and rub it over your lower abdominal area. A warm towel placed over the abdomen would feel nice, too.

Cramp bark *(Viburnum opulus)* is considered a uterine nervine and is the herb of choice for menstrual cramping. Containing one of the same constituents as valerian *(Valeriana officinalis),* valerianic acid, it is both an antispasmodic and a sedative. It combines well with valerian to relieve cramping; both can be found in most products specifically formulated for relieving cramps. If you prefer to make your own remedy, simply combine 1 part valerian root with 1 part cramp bark and follow the instructions for making tinctures in that section. Take 15 drops of the valerian–cramp bark tincture every 15 minutes for up to an hour or until the cramping subsides.

MOTION SICKNESS AND NAUSEA

Once nausea sets in, especially when it's due to motion sickness, it's hard to overcome. There are a few old standby remedies—most women who've been pregnant have heard of or used at least one of them—which help suppress nausea. The first is good old-fashioned soda crackers. The unsalted ones don't work as well, in my opinion. There's something about the salt content that eases an unsettled stomach. In a pinch, my sister has even turned to salt from the little packets on the airplane—and it's worked. If salt intake is not an issue for you, munch on a few Saltines and see if you don't feel better.

Ginger ale is the another suggestion. It works, but not as well as ginger capsules or fresh diced ginger, if you can get it. The recommended amount is 500 milligrams of powdered, capped ginger every two hours until you feel better. I like taking it before I get on a plane or bus and then continuing it as suggested above if motion sickness becomes a problem. My husband chews on approximately 1 teaspoon of diced ginger every hour when he's sailing to remain feeling reasonably well. Flat Coca-Cola also seems to work for nausea, especially if it's due to intestinal flu or a hangover. Take little sips often until the symptoms abate. I have used still-fizzy Coca-Cola in a pinch and it worked for me, but some health care practitioners warn that the carbonation can make matters worse.

Most health food stores carry special acupressure bands for motion sickness. These are $1/2$-inch-wide cloth-covered elastic bands that have a small rubber bump attached to the inside. The bands are worn around the wrist with the "bump" positioned over a specific acupuncture point (the directions on the package show you where). Stimulating the point is thought to reduce nausea. When I was working in at an alternative "pharmacy," a number of customers reported that the bands worked well for them. They particularly liked the idea of not having to ingest anything. Check your local health food store for more information.

Smelling ginger or peppermint essential oil also helps dispel nausea. Try placing a couple of drops of either oil on a tissue. When you feel ill, smell the tissue. This can be continued every 5 minutes (or more often if needed) until you feel better.

MUSCLE ACHES

You may find yourself more active than usual when traveling, especially if you're backpacking, and sore muscles may be the result. Tiger Balm has always been my son's favorite choice for sore, aching muscles, and I actually think he might marry a woman if she were to wear Tiger Balm as a perfume. I like Tiger Liniment, a liquid version of Tiger Balm. You can purchase Tiger Balm in small tins that make it easily portable—but keep it in a plastic bag. Mine got hot, melted all over my small first-aid kit, and created a mess, albeit a good-smelling one. To use either product, just massage it into the sore muscles. Keep in mind that you'll smell strongly of wintergreen, so this remedy might be best used at night. Also, be sure to wash your hands with soap after applying the salve or liniment. You don't want to get this in your eyes or on other sensitive parts of the body.

Homeopathic arnica taken internally will relieve sore muscles as well. Follow the dosage instructions on the bottle of the particular product you buy. Traumeel is a general anti-inflammatory and analgesic homeopathic formulation used externally—just rub it on the sore areas. It's available in most large health food stores. If you can't find it, you might try a local acupuncturist, chiropractor, or homeopath.

MUSCLE OIL BLEND

I like to use this herbal oil blend as a massage oil for relieving pain. I make it myself but have found similar products available for purchase, if you'd prefer not to go to the trouble.

> *1 part St. John's wort oil*
> *1 part dandelion flower oil*
> *1 part arnica oil*
> *lavender essential oil (12 drops for every ounce of the*
>   *herbal oil blend)*

Both St. John's wort and arnica oils may be purchased, but I haven't seen dandelion flower oil available commercially. I make this up myself in spring when dandelions are abundantly in flower. Just ask your neighbors if you might pick their dandelions—they'll be forever grateful, and you'll have great pain-relieving oil. Follow the instructions for making herbal oils in the oils and salves section.

PAIN

There are all kinds of pain—muscle, abdominal, menstrual, joint—and most of them have been covered under the appropriate sections in this book. In general, pain is often due to inflammation of some sort. In addition to using an analgesic—

a substance that relieves pain—it helps to reduce the inflammation. Anti-inflammatories were covered in the section on allergies, but it bears repeating that chamomile, while having a reputation as a gentle, child's herb, is actually a rather strong anti-inflammatory. It may be taken on its own as an infusion (use 1 to 2 teaspoons of dried herb per 1 cup of hot water) or combined with other pain-relieving, anti-inflammatory herbs. Drink several cups of chamomile tea daily when you're treating any inflammation. My favorite anti-inflammatory formula is manufactured by Herb Pharm and called Turmeric/Chamomile Compound. It contains turmeric *(Curcuma longa),* chamomile flower *(Matricaria recutita),* meadowsweet *(Filipendula ulmaria),* licorice root *(Glycyrrhiza glabra),* St. John's wort *(Hypericum perforatum),* and arnica flower *(Arnica montana).* Arnica may be used internally in very small doses, but I do not personally formulate with it.

White willow *(Salix lucida)* bark contains the glycoside salicin, as does meadowsweet, and both are used for their analgesic properties. In fact, it's believed that aspirin was named for meadowsweet's former botanical name, *Spiraea.* White willow bark capsules may be purchased individually, but I prefer the herb in combination with others. Herb Pharm's Willow/Meadowsweet Compound is a good example.

Topical remedies for pain include St. John's wort oil (the wonderful herb that seems to be known only for its anti-depressant properties) arnica oil, and Traumeel. See the section on muscle aches for more information.

POISON OAK, IVY, OR SUMAC

The infamous itching and oozing blisters caused by poison oak, ivy, and sumac are actually a dermatitis (inflammation of the skin) caused by coming in contact with the plant's oils. Not everyone who touches the plants will get it; the contact dermatitis is an allergic reaction—if you aren't allergic to them, nothing happens. Unfortunately, allergies can appear unexpectedly later in life.

Regardless of whether you have come into contact with poison oak, ivy, or sumac, the symptoms and treatments are essentially the same. To begin with, don't use an oil-based product on the rash unless it has stopped oozing and is drying up. Current thought dictates that while the blisters are open and wet, oils will only spread the irritants. Instead, use something to dry up the blisters. If your travels will include being outdoors in areas that are known for poison ivy, oak, or sumac growth, you might consider preparing and taking along some mugwort (*Artemesia vulgaris*) liniment made with apple cider vinegar. It's easy enough to prepare—just follow the instructions for making a tincture in the tinctures and liniments section, but use apple cider vinegar as the menstruum and mugwort for the plant material. A two-week maceration is probably sufficient. Strain and bottle the mugwort vinegar (it's the remedy), and compost your mugwort. Be sure to label the bottle FOR EXTERNAL USE ON POISON OAK, IVY, AND SUMAC. To use it, just wet cotton balls or gauze with the liniment and apply to the rash. It will sting a bit, but it does a great job drying up the blisters. Apply several times a day. If you don't have any mugwort vinegar, just use plain apple cider vinegar. It won't be quite as effective, but it's easily found in most places.

If the itching becomes severe and you find it difficult to rest, you might try any of the calming herbs or tinctures discussed in the sections on anxiety or stress. Kava *(Piper methisticum)*, catnip *(Nepeta cataria)*, chamomile *(Matricaria recutita)*, and valerian (Valeriana officinalis), work well, and can be taken in the same manner described in those two sections. Even drinking 3 to 4 cups of chamomile tea throughout the day will help, easing both distress and inflammation.

A natural remedy that my husband finds very helpful for relieving the itching and pain associated with poison oak is a paste made from bentonite clay and water. Bentonite clay reacts quite differently from other clays when mixed with water—it tends to become gel-like and requires more water than other clays to get the right consistency. To make this paste, place a couple of tablespoons of bentonite clay in a bowl (preferably ceramic) and mix in a bit of water at time. A fork seems to work better than a spoon for breaking up lumps. Once the paste is ready, apply it to the affected areas. Keep in mind that it takes longer to dry than other clays. It may be left on or washed off gently (mugwort vinegar would make a good wash).

Most people find that heat tends to worsen itching. If hot weather does become a problem, cool showers will help relieve the intensity of the itching. Lukewarm baths made with colloidal oats (Aveeno) work as well. The oats are a demulcent and act to soothe inflamed, itchy skin.

If the case of poison ivy, oak, or sumac is severe enough, it can become systemic—which essentially means that the toxins have entered the entire system. That's why folks sometimes find that just as one patch of rash begins to clear up, another one starts in an area of the body that never came into contact with the plants. This can be quite serious and may require medical attention. If you seem to be handling the rash outbreaks all right, Shatoiya de la Tour recommends drinking 3 to 4 cups of sassafras *(Sassafras albidum)* tea throughout the day. Sassafras is considered an alterative and helps the liver cleanse toxins from the blood. It is, however, somewhat difficult on the liver if taken for extended periods and should not be used if you have a compromised liver (hepatitis, cirrhosis, or the like). Since the part of sassafras used is the bark, the tea must be made as a decoction; see the section on teas for more information. Use 1 to 2 teaspoons of sassafras for each cup of water and simmer gently for 15 minutes.

SINUSITIS

An infection and inflammation of the sinuses, sinusitis may occur as a secondary infection resulting from a cold or allergies. Many of the same remedies used to treat congestion can also be used for sinusitis. Because infection is present, herbs with antibacterial properties may be employed as well.

To deliver the plant's properties directly to the sinuses, try herbal steams (see the section on congestion for directions) made with essential oils. Bay, eucalyptus, and rosemary are all good essential oils for sinus problems. If it's impossible to make an herbal steam or if time is short, place a few drops of any of the oils listed above on a tissue and breathe in their aroma. One nice thing about the tissue trick is that you can use it all day long, refreshing it once in a while when the volatile oils have evaporated completely.

Garlic has long been known for its antibacterial and antiviral properties, but what seems less known is that it must be eaten raw to gain those benefits. When garlic is bruised or crushed, it produces a compound called allicin, which is primarily responsible for the plant's antibiotic activity. Cooking seems to destroy garlic's antibacterial properties. Most herbalists suggest eating 1 to 3 cloves of raw garlic three times a day to get the beneficial effect. This is a lot, but if you add it to a salad or crush it raw over spaghetti, it won't seem so difficult. If your travel takes you to any of the Mediterranean countries, finding garlic will be easy indeed.

Goldenseal *(Hydrastis canadensis)* is specific to infections of the sinuses and mucous membranes and is often recommended combined with echinacea (*Echinacea* spp.). If you read Stephen Harrod Buhner's *Herbal Antibiotics,* it will become clear that herbalists do not agree on goldenseal's actual healing attributes. Furthermore, most environmentally aware herbalists also believe goldenseal to be an endangered plant. My feeling is that if you can find a product made with cultivated goldenseal and echinacea, it's worth trying. The recommended dosage for an acute situation is 30 to 45 drops three to five times a day until the symptoms clear. If your sinusitis does not resolve within a week or if fever is present, consult with your health care practitioner.

SORE FEET

What travel doesn't include sore feet? They're a fact of life when you're backpacking, and it's certainly not considered proper wilderness etiquette to complain about them. Most tours consist of long walks interspersed with long bus rides, so you can pretty much bet on a couple of sore pups by the end of the day.

Fortunately, relief is only as far away as your hotel room (or campsite), where you can finally prop your feet up. Elevating your feet will allow lymphatic fluids to drain back toward your heart and will relieve pressure that has built up over the day. After you've had a chance to relax a bit, draw a hot, shallow bath for your feet. Throw in a few drops of lavender or chamomile essential oil for a more relaxing experience, and let your feet soak for at least 10 minutes. If you're camping, heat up some water and fill the dishwashing basin for a nice foot soak—just wash it out afterward!

Once you're done soaking, dry your feet and follow it up with a foot massage. This is nicest if you can get someone else to give it to you, but you can still do it yourself effectively. Peppermint essential oil's invigorating properties feel extra special on sore feet. Pour a bit of unscented lotion or vegetable oil in your hand and add a drop or two of peppermint essential oil. Rub your palms together, distributing the essential oil, and then massage into your feet. While the peppermint oil will at first feel cooling, it's actually warming. It's much like topical applications such as Tiger Balm—people can never agree whether it's hot or cold!

SORE THROAT

Sore throats sometimes are the result of an allergy, but more often than not they herald a cold. They can also mean strep throat or tonsillitis. What should you do if you get one while traveling? A warm saltwater gargle is an old-fashioned remedy that works. Not only soothing and healing, the salt also disinfects the throat. Place 1 to 2 teaspoons of salt in a glass of warm water. (A hotel-sized glass is perfect.) Take a little sip of the warm salt water without swallowing, tilt your head back, and gargle by gently forcing air out through your mouth. If you haven't gargled before, it feels like a whirlpool at the back of your throat. Gargle for about 5 seconds and spit out the water. Continue gargling with the remaining salt water. While you shouldn't swallow the salt water, some is inevitably consumed, so if you have high blood pressure, edema, or any constraints regarding your salt intake you might want to skip this treatment. I find that doing this every couple of hours really helps to clear away any debris from postnasal drip.

Herbal throat lozenges are easy to pack, and sucking on them will relieve some of the pain associated with a sore throat. I prefer the kind with a bit of eucalyptus, since a stuffy nose often accompanies a sore throat. The volatile oils from the eucalyptus help open up the sinuses so it's easier to breathe.

I once complained of frequent sore throats to a massage therapist, who recommended a month's course of sage tea taken twice daily. Her advice turned out to be excellent. Sage *(Salvia officinalis)*, the garden variety, is both antiseptic and antibacterial in action. In addition, it's an astringent, so it's particularly useful for "wet" infections where some mucus is present—namely sore throats. To make sage tea, steep 2 teaspoons of the leaf in 1 cup of hot water for 15 minutes. This may be drunk several times throughout the day or may be used as an excellent gargling solution. In fact, this would be a good substitute for a saltwater gargle if you don't tolerate salt. Sage is a Mediterranean plant but is generally found throughout much of the Western world. If you haven't any in your kit, you might find fresh sage locally— just be certain of your source or comfortable with your identification skills.

I've mentioned Herb Pharm's Echinacea/Propolis Spray several times elsewhere in this book, but sore throats are its primary use. Containing echinacea, propolis, hyssop, sage, and St. John's wort, it relieves pain and helps clear up any infection. It tastes great, too, but then I think most herbs taste good. This might be an acquired taste! To use, spray the back of your throat two or three times and repeat every half hour to two hours, depending on the severity of the sore throat. Finally, remember to drink a lot of liquids. Doing so will keep your throat cool and wet and will flush toxins from your body.

SPLINTERS

These are also called slivers. The main problem with them, obviously, is to remove the offending debris while disturbing the surrounding tissues as little as possible. You'll also want to disinfect the area both before removing the splinter and afterward.

You can remove a splinter with either a needle or tweezers; the needle often works better if there's nothing for a pair of tweezers to grab on to. Whatever implement you decide to use, please be sure to clean it prior to use—either with isopropyl alcohol or a prepackaged disinfectant wipe, or by sterilizing it for few moments with a lit match.

Once the splinter has been removed, clean the area with some sort of disenfectant. I've used echinacea-goldenseal tincture in a pinch, but my favorite is Dr. Kloss's Liniment, made with isopropyl alcohol, goldenseal, cayenne, and myrrh. You can make this yourself; the recipe can be found in Jethro Kloss's book, Back to Eden. Hydrogen peroxide or prepackaged disenfectant wipes can also be used.

If you're unable to remove all of a difficult splinter, a plantain (*Plantago* spp.) poultice will often finish the job. It's best if you can get fresh plantain, but if not, the dried variety will work as well. See the section on abscesses and boils for a detailed description on using poultices. You may find that you need to apply several plantain poultices to extract the splinter; it often works best to leave one on overnight.

SPRAINS

A sprain occurs when the ligaments surrounding a joint are pulled and stretched too far. It's a common injury, especially when walking or hiking. The first thing I give when someone has sprained an ankle—or incurred any other type of injury, for that matter—is 4 drops of Rescue Remedy. A sprain happens suddenly and hurts. Rescue Remedy is perfect for such a situation; it will help calm the individual so other treatments will be more effective.

Next, a dose of homeopathic arnica is required. On my top 10 list, arnica may be used for any kind of traumatic injury to the body and has even been found helpful in reducing postoperative swelling, particularly in dental surgery. Repeat the dose every hour or two for the first twenty-four hours, and then reduce to three to five times a day until the pain and swelling have subsided. I generally purchase homeopathic arnica in the 30x strength.

Be particularly careful if a fracture is suspected. If there's a lot of swelling or heavy bruising, or if the individual cannot walk or bend the injured limb, it's important to get medical attention as soon as possible. If the injury truly seems to be a simple sprain, the current treatment is RICE: "rest, ice, compression, and elevation." Essentially this means that the patient should lie down, raise and ice the injured area, and apply a compress that will reduce swelling. Resting and elevating aren't too difficult to do while traveling, but it might be a bit more involved to accomplish icing and prepare a compress.

If you're anywhere near a grocey store, purchase a couple of bags of frozen peas. Place one over the sprained area to cool the inflammation and reduce swelling. Frozen peas work better than ice because they're smaller and conform to the body more easily— plus they come in their own bag. If you have access to a freezer, you can stick the peas back in and reuse them for icing. Place a thin towel between the skin and the peas (or ice, if you're using an ice bag) to prevent injuring the skin. Keep the bag in place for 15 minutes, take a 30-minute break, and then reapply the peas or ice in this manner until the swelling has decreased, making sure to take a break from the ice every 15 to 30 minutes.

You might want to alternate between ice and a cool compress. Compresses for a sprain should be made with cold water and herbal tinctures and/or essential oils. Any of the following will work: St. John's wort *(Hypericum perforatum)* tincture, arnica *(Arnica montana)* tincture, comfrey *(Symphytum officinale)* tincture, and lavender, rosemary,and marjoram essential oils. If you're using tinctures, add 1 tablespoon to ½ cup of cold water. A few drops of one of the recommended essential oils can also be added. Soak a soft cloth in the cold herbal water, wring it out, and apply it to the sprain. If you have an Ace bandage, you can use it to hold the compress in place by wrapping the area loosely.

At night gently massage a bit of St. John's wort or arnica oil into the injured area. Both are pain relieving and will help the tissues heal. Be sure not to use arnica if the skin is broken.

STRESS

David Hoffmann defines *stress* in his book *An Herbal Guide to Stress Relief* as "the response of the body to a demand." It's an all-encompassing definition and it's true that to the body, getting married—usually thought of as a positive event—feels the same as getting fired. The body doesn't necessarily differentiate between "good" and "bad" when stress is a factor. This section deals briefly with alternative ways to de-stress. There are also many books out on the subject. David Hoffmann's is one; another is Christopher Hobbs's *Stress and Natural Healing*. Both are excellent.

Siberian ginseng *(Eleutherococcus senticosus)* is recommended by Lois Johnson, M.D., as a preventive. She suggests starting it several weeks prior to your trip. Siberian ginseng works as an adaptogen, helping the body adapt to stress. It is not a true ginseng and seems to be milder in action, giving it a wider application. Try 30 to 45 drops three times a day.

Since the body responds to stressors in a physical manner, it helps to respond in the same way when stressed. Exercise is a time-honored treatment. One of the ways the body reacts when stressed is to pump a bunch of adrenaline in the system. It's part of the "fight-or-flight" response, and it's meant to help propel our bodies into action. Usually we just sit around and drink more coffee—not a great idea. Instead, get active. Go for a walk. Use the gym or pool at your hotel. Do calisthenics or yoga in your hotel room.

Once you've worked up a sweat, relaxation is next. If you meditate, you probably already know that it's great for relieving stress. If not, vacation is a good time to start the practice. Simply put on comfortable clothing, place a pillow on the floor next to the wall, and sit cross-legged with your back resting against the wall. Close your eyes and breathe slowly and deeply. As you breathe slowly in, focus on your breath and how it feels as it moves up your nostrils. As you breathe out, focus on the movement your abdomen makes as the breath is released. Whether you focus on your breath or instead repeat a simple, soulful phrase in your mind doesn't matter. It doesn't even matter if your thoughts turn to something else. Simply notice it, smile inwardly, and go back to your original focus. Do this for 20 minutes. Whether you believe it or not, the relaxation this brings to a stressed body is immeasurable.

Valerian *(Valeriana officinalis),* the herbal "vitamin V," is one of my favorite botanical remedies for relieving stress, particularly when the symptoms include insomnia. With this particular plant, you use the root, but due to its high content of volatile oils you prepare the root as an infusion rather than a decoction. Use 1 to 4 teaspoons per 1 cup of hot water and let it infuse for 15 minutes before drinking. Be sure to cover the cup or pot while steeping so that the volatile oils remain where they belong—in the tea. If insomnia is a stress reaction for you, drink a couple of cups of valerian tea an hour or two before bedtime. For some people, valerian is more easily taken as a tincture. See the section on insomnia for dosage amounts and the note regarding valerian's opposing action in certan people.

California poppy *(Eschscholzia californica)* is similar to valerian in that it has hypnotic and sedative actions and is best taken before bedtime. While it's a poppy, it is nonaddictive. One note: The California poppy is the state flower of California. If you happen to be traveling to California during late spring or summer and are out and among these beautiful golden flowers, don't pick any for your tea. It's illegal to pick them in the wild in California. Read John Steinbeck's description of spring in the Californian foothills in the first few pages of *East of Eden* to understand why. They are simply stunning! California poppy can be used as a tincture; take 30 to 45 drops at night.

Lemon balm *(Melissa officinalis)* is wonderful taken as a tea because it has a lovely, mild lemony flavor. In addition to being a relaxant, it has a mild carminative action, which makes it doubly useful if part of your stress is due to indigestion. To prepare lemon balm tea, use 2 to 4 teaspoons per 1 cup of hot water. Let it steep for 10 minutes before drinking.

I like using lavender *(Lavandula angustifolia)* best in its essential oil form, in a bath or on a tissue, but the herb, not the essential oil, can also be taken as a tincture or standard infusion. If you're using a tincture, try 30 to 45 drops three times a day. A tea may be made of 2 to 4 teaspoons of the lavender flowers per 1 cup of hot water. Let it steep for 15 minutes before drinking; as when preparing a valerian infusion, make sure to cover the cup or pot to retain lavender's volatile oils. If you happen to be in Provence in summer, indulge in a picnic among the fields of lavender. The scent alone will leave everyone blissful.

If you can, book a massage. If you're on vacation, you deserve one, and if you're on a business trip you *really* deserve one! Massage therapy is one of the best ways to relieve stress. It helps the body move stress-related toxins through the lymph system (drink lots of water afterward), is soothing to the soul, and feels incredible. Ask specifically for an aromatherapy treatment and let them know you want to de-stress. If they don't have an aromatherapist on staff, take along some lavender essential oil and ask them to add a few drops to the massage oil they plan to use on you. Finally, I think about what my mother always told me when I was particularly upset about something or other: "This too shall pass."

SWOLLEN FEET OR ANKLES

Often the result of air and auto travel, as well as long excursions exploring your destination, swollen feet and ankles can put an end to any comfort you might have had up to that point. To avoid the problem, don't eat foods that you know cause water retention. Excess salt is often a culprit. Make sure to keep your body hydrated. Paradoxically, drinking a lot of water works as a mild diuretic—it helps your body rid itself of excess water. Try to elevate your feet as often as possible. This isn't often possible in a cramped airplane, but if you're fortunate enough to be on a half-full flight, take advantage of any extra seating to get your feet up. Lois Johnson, M.D., recommends hourly calf stretches. Simply flex your foot at the ankle repeatedly for about 30 seconds. Repeat with the other foot. This little exercise helps to move fluids through the lymphatic system, relieving buildup in your feet. If the inevitable happens, try a witch hazel spritzer.

Witch Hazel Spritzer

Spritzers are magic in a bottle. You can make them up and use them for all sorts of things. Fill a small 2- to 4-ounce spray-pump bottle (plastic is best for traveling, but glass will do as well) with witch hazel extract. Add 20 to 40 drops of either peppermint or lavender essential oil, cap, and shake. Take this spritzer bottle with you on your travels and spray your feet with it when they become swollen. Witch hazel is an astringent and will temporarily tighten the tissues of your feet. Peppermint essential oil is cooling, invigorating, and analgesic—it will work gently on any pain accompanying tired, swollen feet. Lavender essential oil is relaxing, smells refreshing, and also has mild analgesic activity. Use whichever suits your spirit, and nose, the best. A wonderful feature of this preparation is that you can spray it directly over your nylons. The witch hazel evaporates quickly, so there's no need to take your pantyhose off. Socks will have to be removed, of course! Another plus is the effect of essential oils on stale, smelly feet.

TRAUMA

It isn't pleasant to imagine the kinds of traumatic experiences you might have while traveling. It's also true that the severity of trauma varies widely; what might be traumatic for one person is simply an inconvenience for another. I'm hoping that you encounter nothing more than inconvenience in your travels.

When trauma is an issue, though, Rescue Remedy should be your first choice. There are some who feel that no matter what the ailment or problem, Rescue Remedy is useful. It certainly won't hurt. That's why you'll often hear flower essence practitioners refer to Rescue Remedy as the "first-aid kit in a bottle." Also remember that illness or injury is often traumatic for those involved in caring for the individual or who might have seen an accident take place. These folks should take Rescue Remedy as well. The standard dosage is 4 drops under the tongue. This can be repeated at 15-minute intervals for severe trauma, or three to five times a day for a situational inconvenience. One trick is to put 12 drops of Rescue Remedy into a bottle filled with water and drink it throughout the day if you know that the whole day is going to be difficult. A perfect example is air travel. Not only will drinking from a water bottle laced with Rescue Remedy make the flight more pleasant, but you'll be hydrating yourself simultaneously. Anytime you make a compress, add a few drops of Rescue Remedy.

My second choice is lavender essential oil. Simply place a few drops on a tissue and give it to the person who is experiencing trauma. Like Rescue Remedy, it may be beneficial for everyone involved, so pass those lavender tissues around. Here's to a trauma-free trip!

YEAST INFECTIONS

Yeast infections are caused by the overgrowth of an organism called *Candida albicans,* which lives in the vagina. Formerly called *Monilia,* this organism is both a fungus and a yeast, depending on when it's examined. *Candida* and other organisms are present in all healthy vaginas, but under certain conditions they will quickly multiply and cause the symptoms associated with a yeast infection.

Vaginas are normally self-cleansing; they do so by secreting mucus from the vaginal walls. This will result in small amounts of discharge, which may change in both amount and color throughout the monthly cycle. This discharge is entirely normal. However, one of the signs of a vaginal infection is an atypical discharge, meaning one that's different in color, amount, or odor than what's usual. A yeast infection will produce a white, curdlike discharge with a yeasty, foul odor. Often there's itchiness present, as well as soreness and inflammation around the vagina. Sexual intercourse can be quite painful at this time.

What causes a yeast infection? As noted above, the offending organism lives, in check, in all healthy vaginas. But a number of situations can lead to rapid overgrowth of the organism. Weakness in the immune system, caused by stress or by allowing yourself to become generally run down, will allow the organism to multiply unchecked. Changing your diet to one of rich foods with concentrated amounts of sugar and animal proteins can provide an appropriate environment for *Candida* overgrowth. Sexual intercourse can also have an unfortunate effect in that the presence of semen raises the vagina's pH and causes it to become more alkaline, creating a more hospitable environment for the *Candida*.

Travel and holidays abroad often create all three of the conditions noted above. Long, cramped trips on an airplane supplied with recycled, stale air and little sleep put undue stress on a body. A vacation just isn't a vacation if you don't get to indulge in a few of your favorite foods—especially those that aren't "good" for you. And if you're lucky enough to travel with your partner, you might find that you're both more amorous than usual.

Fortunately, there are remedies for the situation that aren't necessarily difficult to obtain, even in the remotest of locations. Also, if you're prone to yeast infections, it's wise to be prepared. You might want to make up a few of the following preparations and take them with you, especially if you'll be backpacking and away from civilization. In addition, it helps to avoid sexual intercourse until the infection has resolved itself—you probably won't feel much like lovemaking anyway. Don't wash with soap;

cool, pure water is best in this situation. To help keep the vaginal tissues dry, dust with cornstarch morning and night. Forget about wearing tight-fitting pants and try to wear cotton underwear—or at least underwear with a cotton crotch. Choose whole foods if possible, and avoid or limit your intake of alcohol, coffee, black tea, and sugar.

Yogurt

One of the easiest and most soothing remedies for a vaginal yeast infection is plain, unsweetened, unflavored yogurt. You should be able to find it pretty much anywhere. There are several ways to use the yogurt. First, you can eat it daily as a preventive measure if you know you're susceptible, although you really want to get the yogurt straight to the source. To do this, soak a tampon (made from organic cotton, if possible, but certainly don't stress about it if these aren't available—any kind will do) in the yogurt and then insert it into the vagina as best you can. You'll need to use your fingers; an applicator will be useless at this point. This is a messy procedure and, once it's done, you'll need to lie down and stay put for a while. Be sure to put a towel or some kind of protective covering underneath you. If you can leave the tampon in overnight, so much the better, but even an hour or two will help. Upon arising, remove the tampon and wash well with cool water only. You may find that you need to do this once or twice a day until the infection clears up.

Another method that's less troublesome—although it's also somewhat less effective, because the yogurt doesn't get inside well—is to apply the yogurt directly to the vaginal area. Be sure to coat all vaginal tissues. Again, you will need to lie down and rest, which can be medicine in itself. Our bodies have a great number of ways to tell us to rest. The yogurt will cool and soothe the inflamed tissues and should feel wonderful once you're able to relax.

Tea Tree Douche

I must preface this section by saying that I've never tried a tea tree douche. I know women who have, and they've told me that while it stings, it can be very effective. The treatment requires having a douche bag at your disposal, something you aren't likely to pack when traveling. But they aren't uncommon in Europe and you should be able to find one if you decide to try it. There are a number of variations on the following douche recipe; this is a pared-down version (simpler for travel) of one suggested by Kathi Keville in her book *Herbs for Health and Healing*.

Put 6 drops of tea tree essential oil in 3 cups of warm water. Add this to a douche bag and shake well. This combination should be used once a day. Kathi recommends not using it for longer than five days.

Salt Bath

Stress exacerbates yeast conditions, so any relief from the wear and tear of traveling is useful. A warm bath will facilitate relaxation and, coupled with a cup or two of sea salt, will help control a yeast infection. Finding sea salt shouldn't be a problem in most locations.

To take a salt bath, fill a tub with warm water—not too hot—and add 2 cups of sea salt. Five to 7 drops of lavender essential oil thrown in for good measure will increase the bath's relaxing properties. Soak in the tub for 10 to 15 minutes. Upon emerging, dry yourself completely, especially the vulva. It helps—and feels good—to gently dry your pubic area with a hair dryer set on cool or warm. Dust with cornstarch if you have it.

Tincture

An effective internal remedy that you can use in conjunction with any of the external treatments above is the old traveler's standby—echinacea-goldenseal tincture. Certainly this item does double duty and more. At the first sign of infection, begin taking 30 to 45 drops of the tincture every two hours. As symptoms wane, you can reduce the intake of the tincture to 30 to 45 drops three times a day. Remember to continue taking the reduced dosage several days a week after the symptoms are gone.

Yeast infections can be difficult to eradicate. While the above remedies work well, if your infection gets worse or continues after you return home, it would be wise to consult your health care practitioner.

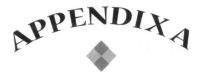

APPENDIX A

CHILDREN'S DOSAGES

If you want to learn about which herbs are appropriate for children's minor ailments, I recommend reading *Kids, Herbs, and Health: A Parent's Guide to Natural Remedies* by Linda B. White, M. D., and Sunny Mavor and *Rosemary Gladstar's Herbal Remedies for Children's Health* by Rosemary Gladstar. As I mentioned earlier in the book, not all herbs that are safe for adults are gentle enough for children, so be sure to gather information before your trip.

There are a number of different ways to determine appropriate dosages of remedies for children. The following guidelines are specifically for the administering of herbal formulations. Young's Rule uses age to determine dosage, while Clark's Rule uses weight. Since a child's weight is so individual and often seems to have little to do with age (one child may weigh 65 pounds at the age of eleven and another may weigh 110), weight is probably the more accurate yardstick. Supplement dosage should be determined in consultation with your health care practitioner.

- **Young's Rule.** The child's age divided by 12 plus the age will give the approximate child's dose. Example: A six-year-old child.

  $6 \div (12 + 6) = 6 \div 18 = .33$ **or 1/3 of the adult dose**

- **Clark's Rule.** The child's weight (in pounds) divided by 150 (average weight in pounds for an adult) will give the approximate child's dose. Example: An 80-pound child.

  $80 \div 150 = .53$ **or $1 \div 2$ of the adult dose**

- **If you're using kilos, Clark's Rule can be restated:** The child's weight (in kilos) divided by 70 (average weight in kilos for an adult) will give the approximate child's dose. Example: A child weighing 25 kilos.

  $25 \div 70 = .4$ **or $2 \div 5$ of the adult dose.**

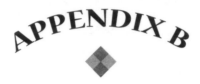

RESOURCES

CONTAINERS

For making your own herbal remedies, the following companies offer reasonable prices on bottles, jars, and other packaging items.

SKS Bottle and Packaging, Inc.
3 Knabner Road
Mechanicville, NY 12118
Tel: 518-899-7488
Fax: 800-810-0440
www.sks-bottle.com

Sunburst Bottle Company
5710 Auburn Boulevard #7
Sacramento, CA 95841
Tel: 916-348-5576
Fax: 916-348-3803
E-mail: sunburst@cwo.com
www.sunburstbottle.com

EDUCATIONAL PROGRAMS

California School of Herbal Studies
P.O. Box 39
Forestville, CA 95436
Tel: 707-887-7457
www.cshs.com

Sage Mountain
P.O. Box 420
E. Barre, VT 05649
Tel: 802-479-9825
Fax: 802-476-3722
www.sagemountain.com
Rosemary Gladstar's onsite apprenticeships and correspondence course

Shatoiya and Rick de la Tour
3500 Fir Mountain Road
Hood River, OR 97031
Write for information

Rocky Mountain Center for Botanical Studies, Inc.
2639 Spruce Street
P.O. Box 19254
Boulder, Colorado 80308-2254
Tel: 303-442-6861
Fax: 303-442-6294
www.herbschool.com

ESSENTIAL OILS

The Essential Oil Company
1719 S.E. Umatilla
Portland, OR 97202
Tel: 503-872-8735
Fax: 800-825-2885
E-mail: office@essentialoil.com
www.essentialoil.com

Liberty Natural Products, Inc.
8120 S.E. Stark Street
Portland, OR 97215
Tel: 800-289-8427
www.libertynatural.com

FLOWER ESSENCES

Alaskan Flower Essence Project
P.O. Box 1369
Homer, Alaska 99603
Tel: 907-235-2188
Fax: 907-235-2777
Orders: 800-545-9309
E-mail: info@alaskanessences.com
www.alaskanessences.com

Nelson Bach
Wilmington Technology Park
100 Research Drive
Wilmington, MA 01887
Tel: 800-314-BACH (orders)
Tel: 800-334-0843 (education)

Woodland Essence
P.O. Box 206
Cold Brook, NY 13324
Tel: 315-845-1515
Tree, Shrub, and Forest Floor Flower Essences

HERBS AND
HERBAL PRODUCTS

Avena Botanicals
20 Mill Street
Rockland, ME 04865
Tel: 207-594-0694
www.avenaherbs.com

Dry Creek Herb Farm
14245 Edgehill Lane
Auburn, CA 95603
Tel: 530-888-0889
Tel: 530-888-0839
www.drycreekherbfarm.com

Healing Spirits
9198 St. Rt. 415
Avoca, NY 14809
Tel: 5607-566-2701
Excellent quality organic and wildcrafted herbs—must buy by
the pound

Jean's Greens
119 Sulphur Spring Road
Norway, NY 13416
Tel: 315-845-6500
www.jeansgreens.com

Mountain Rose Herbs
20818 High Street
North San Juan, CA 95960
Tel: 800-879-3337
Fax: 530-292-9138
www.botanical.com/mtrose

StarWest Botanicals
11253 Trade Center Drive
Rancho Cordova, CA 95742
Tel: 800-800-4372 or 916-853-9354
Fax: 916-853-9673
E-mail: sales-w@starwest-botanicals.com

ORGANIZATIONS

The Flower Essence Society
P.O. Box 459
Nevada City, CA 95959
Tel: 800-548-0075 or 916-265-9163
www.flowersociety.org

Herb Research Foundation
1007 Pearl Street, Suite 200
Boulder, CO 80302
Tel: 303-449-2265
www.herbs.org

National Center for Homeopathy
801 N. Fairfax Street, Suite 306
Alexandria, VA 22314
Tel: 877-624-0613 or 703-548-7790
Fax: 703-548-7792
www.homeopathic.org

WEB SITES

www.mothernature.com
Natural products and educational information
www.drweil.com
Dr. Andrew Weil's Web site

www.yahoo.com
Look under "Health>Alternative Medicine" for an excellent
selection of alternative health sites

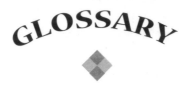

GLOSSARY

alterative: an herb or substance affecting the underlying systems of the body and causing positive change in the overall health of the individual; sometimes known as a blood or liver cleanser

analgesic: an herb or substance that relieves pain

anodyne: an herb or substance that relieves pain

antitussive: an herb or substance that relieves coughing

astringent: an herb or substance that causes the tissues to contract

carminative: an herb or substance that promotes the secretion of bile, enhancing digestion and relieving flatulence

demulcent: an herb or substance that is soothing and healing to the tissues; often mucilaginous in texture

156

febrifuge: an herb or substance that reduces fever

hemostatic: an herb or substance that stops bleeding

hypnotic: an herb or substance that promotes sleep

nervine: an herb or substance that has a direct effect on the nerves, either as a stimulant, sedative, or nourisher

regencrative: an herb or substance that promotes regeneration of a particular tissue or system

rubifacient: an herb or substance that increases blood flow to the surface of the skin causing a temporary reddening and possible irritation

styptic: an herb or substance that stops bleeding, usually through an astringent action

tonic: an herb or substance that may be used for long periods of time and that promotes overall health and well-being; a restorative

vulnerary: an herb or substance that promotes the healing of wounds

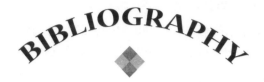

BIBLIOGRAPHY

Balch, James F., Phyllis A. Balch. *Prescription for Nutritional Healing.* Garden City Park, N.Y.: Avery, 1990.

Buhner, Stephen Harrod. *Herbal Antibiotics.* Pownal, Vt.: Storey Books, 1999.

Caperonis, Daphna. "Beat the Cold." *Natural Health,* October 2000, 95.

Cech, Richo. *Making Plant Medicine.* Williams, Oreg.: Horizon Herbs, 2000.

Crawford, Amanda McQuade. *Herbal Remedies for Women.* Rocklin, Calif.: Prima Publishing, 1997.

Gladstar, Rosemary. *The Science and Art of Herbology.* Barre,Vt.: Sage, 2000.

———. *Rosemary Gladstar's Herbal Remedies for Children's Health.* Pownal, Vt.: Storey Books, 1999.

———. *Herbal Healing for Women.* New York: Fireside, 1993.

Grieve, Mrs. M. *A Modern Herbal.* 2 vols. 1931. Reprint, New York: Dover Publications, 1981.

Harrar, Sari, and Sara Alstshul O'Donnell. *The Woman's Book of Healing Herbs.* Emmaus, Penn.: Rodale Press, 1998.

Hobbs, Christopher. *Natural Liver Therapy.* Capitola, Calif.: Botanica Press, 1996.

————. *Stress and Natural Healing.* Loveland, Colo.: Botanica Press, 1997.

Hoffmann, David. *The New Holistic Herbal.* Rockport, Mass.: Element, 1992.

————. *An Herbal Guide to Stress Relief.* Rochester, Vt.: Healing Arts Press, 1991.

Howard, Judy. *The Bach Flower Remedies Step by Step.* Essex, England: Saffron Walden, C. W. Daniel Company, 1997.

Kaminski, Patricia, and Richard Katz. *Flower Essence Repertory.* Nevada City, Calif.: The Flower Essence Society, 1994.

Kemper, Kathi J. *The Holistic Pediatrician.* New York: HarperPerennial, 1996.

Keville, Kathi. *Herbs for Health and Healing.* Emmaus, Penn.: Rodale Press, 1996.

Keville, Kathi, and Mindy Green. *Aromatherapy: A Complete Guide to the Healing Art.* Freedom, Calif.: The Crossing Press, 1995.

Moore, Michael. *Medicinal Plants of the Pacific West.* Santa Fe: Red Crane Books, 1993.

Shealy, C. Norman. *The Illustrated Encyclopedia of Natural Remedies.* Boston, Mass.: Element Books, 1998.

Smith, Ed. *Therapeutic Herb Manual.* N. p., 1997.

Soule, Deb. *The Roots of Healing.* New York: Carol Publishing Group, 1995.

Tierra, Michael. *The Way of Herbs.* New York: Pocket Books, 1990.

Tisserand, Robert B. *The Art of Aromatherapy.* Rochester, Vt.: Healing Arts Press, 1977.

Vogel, H. C. A. *The Nature Doctor.* New Canaan, Conn.: Keats Publishing,1991.

Weil, Andrew. *Natural Health, Natural Medicine.* Boston: Houghton Mifflin Company, 1990.

White, Linda B. "Herbal Tricks for Easing Anxiety." *Herbs for Health,* Sept.–Oct. 2000, 35.

———. "Fending Off Colds and Flu." *Herbs for Health,* Sept.–Oct. 1999, 58.

White, Linda B., and Sunny Mavor. *Kids, Herbs, and Health: A Parent's Guide to Natural Remedies.* Loveland, Colo.: Interweave Press, 1998.

Wood, Matthew. *The Book of Herbal Wisdom.* Berkeley, Calif.: North Atlantic Books, 1997.

Worwood, Valerie Ann. *The Complete Book of Essential Oils and Aromatherapy.* San Rafael, Calif.: New World Library, 1991.